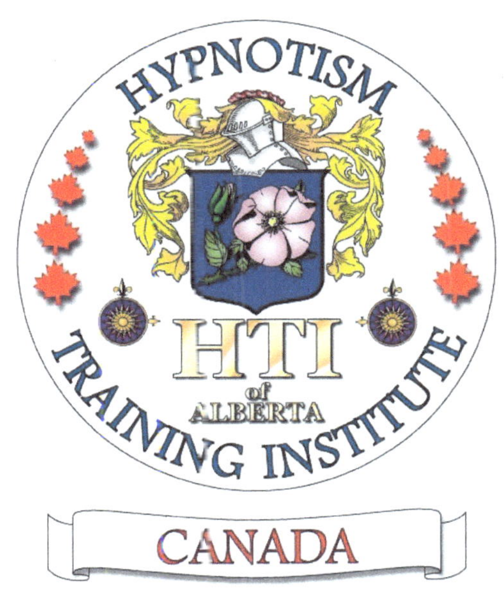

Hypnosis 204

Healing With Hypnotherapy

By Anny J. Slegten

Healing With Hypnotherapy
Anny Slegten
Published by
Kimberlite Publishing House
www.kimberlitePublishingHouse.com

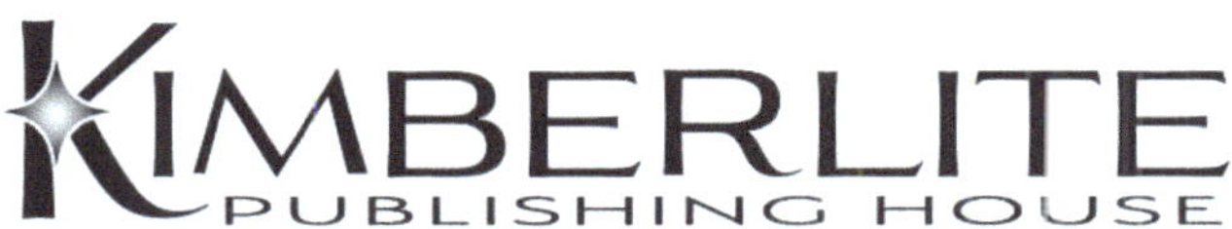

The author of this book does not dispense medical advice or prescribe the use of any technique as a form of treatment for physical, emotional, mental, spiritual or medical problems without the advice of a physician, either directly or indirectly. The intent of the author is only to offer information of a general nature to help you in your quest for physical, mental, emotional and spiritual wellbeing.

In the event you use any of the information in this book for yourself, which is your right, the author and the publisher assume no responsibility for your actions.

ISBN: 978-1-7752489-8-9

School Coat of Arms designed by Boomer Stralak
Book layout by Colin Christopher *www.colinchristopher.com*
Book cover and Kimberlite Logo designed by Marietta Miller
www.execugraphx.com

The Kimberlite-Diamond Connection

Kimberlite is a rock type that was first categorized over a 100 years ago based on descriptions of the diamond-bearing pipes of Kimberley, South Africa.

Kimberlites are the mechanism by which diamonds are brought to the surface.

Kimberlitic rocks are the most important primary source of diamonds and the main rock type in which significant diamond deposits have been found so far.

Anny is familiar with many rocks and minerals as her husband was raised around quarries, and later worked in several mines in Canada.

Therefore, it was natural for Anny to choose kimberlite as an analogy to the soul residing within our body – as a diamond within the kimberlite.

A Picture Is Worth A Thousand Words

Did you notice the little 7 ½ cm (3 inches) clay pot, gracing the cover of this book?

What does that have to do with regression therapy and past lives?

Well, this little clay pot was returned to me in 1992. When I saw it, I recognized it, knew it was mine and what I was using it for.

I instantly burst into tears as I found myself in a past life. I was back there, reliving that time of so long ago.

Wonder what is the story behind the little clay pot?

I will tell you in class…

Anny

Welcome to

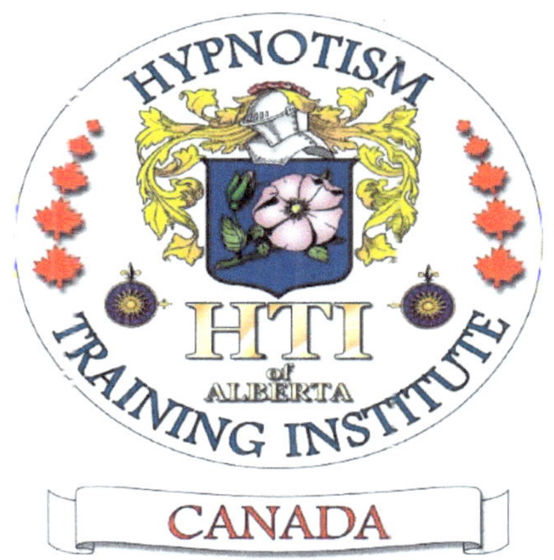

HYP 204 – Healing With Hypnotherapy

This book belongs to:

Name ______________________________

Mailing Address ______________________________

____

City or Town ______________________________

Province/State ____________________ Postal Code/Zip ________

Country ______________________________

Telephone Home (___) __________ Work (___) __________

Instructor's Name: ***Anny Slegten***

Today's Date: ______________________________

Table Of Contents

A Note From Anny

The design and development of the Course Material required the investment of substantial effort, time and money and is only intended for the participants of HYP 204, Healing With Hypnotherapy.

Understand that the experiences derived from attending this course is a private and personal experience for each participant. As such please do respect the confidentiality of all participants and their remarks and actions and keep all such information private and confidential.

As a result, I am counting on you do your part at keeping this course environment safe and secure for all participants.

Enjoy!

Your Notes

Anny's Teaching

Let Us Have A Review

Please read these three questions. As the course unfold, write down your answers.

The answers will be reviewed by the end of the course.

Enjoy!

1. As you are reviewing what you have learned so far, as a hypnotherapist, what is the common denominator when doing hypnosis and doing hypnotherapy?

2. When doing a session, what is the difference between a hypnosis session and a hypnotherapy session?

3. What is the result for you personally?
   How is your relationship to life?

Your Notes

Anny's Teaching

Past Life Information

To understand our essence as human beings, compare your body to a car and your soul as the driver of that car. Notice that the maker of the car tempts you to buy it by advertising and so forth. However, it is the buyer who is the owner of that car and usually drives it too.

A woman, our future mother, is in the cycle of offering a body to a soul; it is the soul who decides to take the opportunity to have a physical experience. Understanding that our reason to come back is always to put closure on an unfinished business, the last thought as we die, we realize we chose our mother for *our* good, nobody else's!

Reincarnation, our physical manifestation, our physical experience this time around starts at conception as we begin the cycle of life, having chosen the mother, the country and all that is attached to the whole. One can say we take on a package deal with the idea to shake off an unfinished business.

What is that unfinished business, our Karma?

Life is circular until having resolved the issue that is sitting heavily on our shoulders, and when going from one past life to the previous one, to the one before, and we can go on and on about it, we realize the issue we are encountering is always the same one, under different coats we are wearing.

Wanting to know what you came back to resolve is rather easy: Check your life and notice the re-occurring patterns. One can tell. It is like turning in a circle until one gets it right.

Your Notes

Anny's Teaching

Sometimes the client does not know who they are when finding themselves in a past life. I then ask them to check their feet and ask them to describe them. This usually gives the client an idea of their location, age and gender.

When a client gets into a past life, it is important to make them go to the point of death and make the person aware of what is on their mind. Then, once out of their body, to look back, ask what they perceive, and what is on their mind.

Whatever it is, is usually what will make them come back to atone, to shake off. As they release their spirit from their body, sometimes they know their body released their soul, sometimes they are not aware of it and wonder what happened and where they are, feeling lost.

There are 2 stages after death:

First, earthbound, the planning stage, in limbo, purgatory or whatever you call it.

The second stage is going THROUGH a very beautiful soft white light, regardless of religion or the lack of it.

The decision to leave the first stage and move forward is a very personal decision. To do so, they must go *through* the light to go to their house, to heaven or hell, depending on their conscience.

To make sure my clients are getting the two sides of that past life experience, I make a point asking them to go to the highlight of that life and the most enjoyable time in that life. Sometimes, I also ask my client – still in that particular life – "what have you learned?" The answer is most revealing of what the Karma is all about.

Just like dreams, some people believe in the messages of a dream, some people do not believe in them and disregard them, I do understand that.

Your Notes

Anny's Teaching

Some people do not believe in past life.

Sometimes it is the client, sometimes it is the hypnotherapist.

Believing in it or not believing in it is not the point. What counts is to help the person to heal whatever has to be healed and put closure on whatever they wanted to put closure on: the reason you are receiving these instructions.

Your Notes

Anny's Teaching

More On Anchoring

Anchoring can be useful in many cases, one of them is to expand the finesse of a language to an other language, or a skill to another skill.

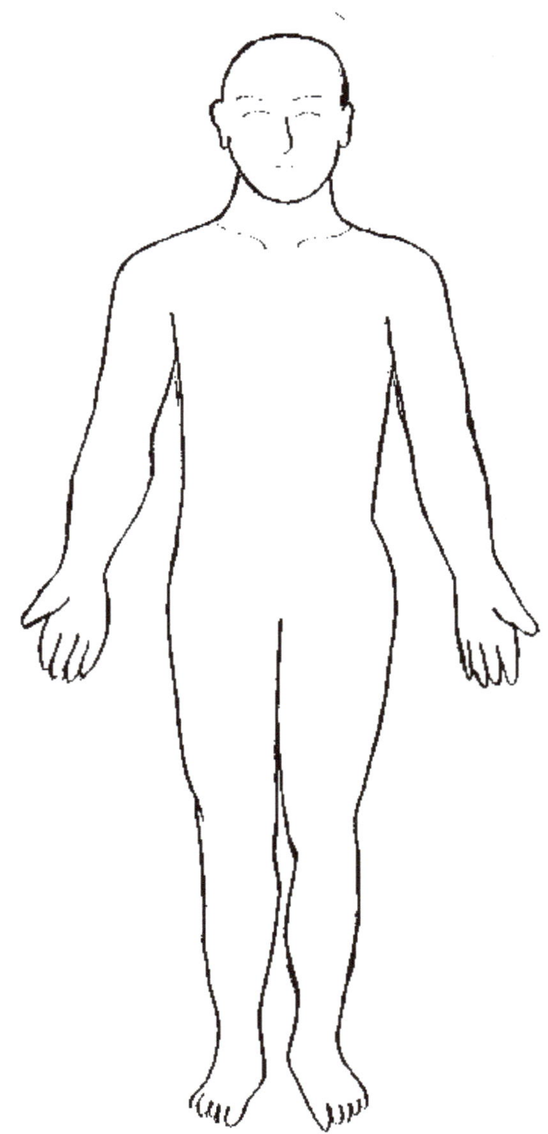

Your Notes

Anny's Teaching

Dream Arm

A Neuro Linguistic Programming Technique (N.L.P.)

A Technique to improve task performance.

One arm up over head.

1. Imagine the person you admire at being successful in the field you want to be as good in.

That person is very successful and very good at what you want to be doing yourself.

"See" that person as if you were watching him or her, as in a movie. As you are watching the movie, allow your arm to slowly come down.

You will be at the end of the movie when your hand touches your leg.

2. Repeat: Arm up this time put yourself in place of the admired person, doing the task successfully.

As you are watching yourself in the movie, allow your arm to slowly come down.

You will be at the end of the movie when your hand touches your leg.

3. Repeat again, arm up: This time, the cameras are on you and you have the pleasure of doing the task with ease.

As you are enjoying performing the task of your choice, allow your arm to slowly come down.

Your hand will touch your leg at the end of the task.

Your Notes

Anny's Teaching

Going Into Someone's Head

Another "Tool" For The Toolbox

Introduction

There was a question about going into somebody's head to see through their eyes.

So you are going to experience that for yourself.

I would like you to think of somebody that you do not understand. There is something there that you do not understand and because of that the relationship is not that great. What is happening? You really want to understand. You want to understand their point of view and you want them to understand your point of view. Very enlightening by the way!

Suggestion

I would like you to take a deep breath and as you exhale find yourself in a place that suggests relaxation to you, and close your eyes. Find yourself there and tell yourself that with each exhale you become more and more relaxed. More and more at peace. Letting all your cares fade away, fade away, fade away, fade away.

As I am asking for our protection and our well-being and I say, "God, please allow only good things to come to us. And for this blessing we give thanks."

And now, you ask to be placed into the protection of your very own light, your very own light, your spark of life. It is like a mini sun in your chest. Some people can see it, some people can feel it, some people simply know it is there. That light of yours, that very beautiful light of yours, let it shine, let it shine, let it shine throughout every cell of your body, throughout your aura, cleansing your body, cleansing your aura, strengthening your

Your Notes

Anny's Teaching

body, strengthening your aura, extending itself at one arm's length above you, beneath you, on each side of you, in front of you and behind you and mentally repeat with me:

"This is my body, this is my space, only light can come to me, only light can come from me, only my light can be here.

And as you take a slow deep breath and exhale find yourself in front of the person that you really want to understand. There is something about it, and you cannot understand the person, and it is obvious that the person does not understand you neither. This is obvious to you.

So, as you are in front of that person, ask for permission to get into their head, explaining to them that you are going to also give them that permission and then respectfully get into their head. And look around.

You are going to find out all kinds of things that are going on in that head. And trust what comes to your awareness and trust it completely, trust it.

What is happening there? Look in all the nooks and crannies, at everything. Look at it. You will find their faults and also the good side of them, you are going to see their skills, everything, whatever it is that you really want to understand.

Look around and find it out. If it is not bright enough turn the light on. Look inside of them.

And then, put yourself behind their eyes. And look at you through their eyes. How do they see you? Notice that! According to them, what are you reflecting to them, whatever it is? You look at them: they look at you through their own eyes. And, as you are looking there, you see how they perceive you.

That is right.

And then, when you get that information about their forte, what they are good at, what they are not good at, and most of all, their skills, their

Your Notes

Anny's Teaching

abilities, what they feel, not sure about, whatever. And, most of all, how they perceive you.

And when you have that information, you are going to stay in a deep trance, as you open your eyes, and write down that information.

That is right. Write it down as you stay in a very deep state of relaxation.

(Pause)

And when you are done, put the pen down, and go right back into that very special quality of relaxation that is so comfortable, and very familiar to you too.

(Pause)

And, as you take a slow, deep breath and exhale, now you graciously get out of that person's head.

And now, allow that person to come into your head. So that they look in all the nooks and crannies, and then what you are hiding, what is obvious, the whole thing.

And you are very much aware of what they are realizing by getting to know you that way. Let that person that comes into your head there, look around and turn the lights on, if it is necessary, it must be crystal clear, crystal clear.

They will know what you are good at, what you are not good at, everything about you, and you are going to become very much aware of how that person sees you, as they are checking you out.

Your Notes

Anny's Teaching

And, then, as you take a slow deep breath and exhale, that person is getting behind your eyes, and sees themself the way you see them. You are going to become very much aware of how that person perceives you. Crystal clear, whether you like it or not. Crystal clear. How is that person perceiving you?

And then, as you take a slow, deep breath and exhale, only when you got that information, crystal clear, about what that person and how they perceive you as they are looking at you, and also what they found out about you, everything about you, as they did visit your head, and then you will take a slow deep breath and as you exhale you will open your eyes and write down what you got, the information you got, staying in a very deep trance.

(Pause)

And as you take a slow, deep breath and exhale, you will have them graciously leave your head and just allow yourself to go deeper and deeper in that very special quality of relaxation.

As I am asking your subconscious mind, open and very receptive to the suggestions you are receiving now to help you clarify the situation, to clarify it, and giving you the information or the solutions, or whatever else that you want, by having understood how the other person views you, and understands you, and thinks you are, and how you perceive and think how they are.

I am asking your subconscious mind, to give that information to you, in a most comforting way. Comforting and beneficial way, to resolve whatever has to be resolved, hear whatever has to be heard, improve whatever has to be improved, so that all this or something even better now manifests itself in your attitude, your behaviour, your life, your relationship with that person, in a most delightful way.

Your Notes

Anny's Teaching

And the benefits of this exercise will stay with you for hours, days, weeks, months and years to come, much to your surprise and delight.
That is right.

And when everything is in sync within you, there is quite a deep understanding there, when everything within you feels comfortable about what you found out, knowing that you will get more information at a most unexpected time, only then will you be able to open your eyes, feeling refreshed, relaxed, renewed, at peace with yourself and with the world around you.

Your Notes

Anny's Teaching

Tibetan Energy

To remove scars or to help damaged tissues or bone(s) to heal faster.

This is to shatter the energy line that “holds” the illness, scars or injury within the physical body. It is very much like a technique I learned during a weekend course given by a Shaman. It is how to break the energy connection between the physical and emotional bodies.

This weekend course name was “The Apprentice Sorcerer” and the Psychologist friend of mine who was hosting this course told me I was the first one to sign up for the course.
During that course, the Shaman was using the North American indigene way of doing this, with drums, rattles, eagle feathers, chants, and dances. I may explain this during class if the Shaman’s method is also of interest to you.

Now, back to the Tibetan Energy.

Using your whole hand (or if the area is very small, two fingers) stroke the area that is sensitive in a figure "8" pattern. Draw it along the pain so that the "8" looks like an "8" and then try drawing it across the pain (or scar) So that the "8" appears to be lying down. This is called a "Lazy 8". One way will feel better to you. You can touch the skin (or the clothing over the area) if it feels right to do so, or you can float the "8" in the air above the pain, because it would be too sensitive to touch, as in a burn, or inappropriate to touch. You can be as much as 3" away from the area.

Keep drawing the figure "8" till you get bored or till the pain subsides, and until you or your friend sighs deeply, which is a way of releasing the stuck energy of pain.

Your Notes

Anny's Teaching

This technique hastens healing as well as relieving pain. Teach it to your children so they can relieve the skinned knees and bruises themselves. You can do figure "8's" on yourself or on others.

As I am recollecting this, we may achieve the same things in different ways. It is like re-inventing the wheel over and over again.

The most important aspect of it all is understanding we broaden our horizon when honoring other cultures as well as other people's teachings and life experiences and adjust our way of doing what we do to the beliefs and cultures of the person we are dealing with.

Your Notes

Anny's Teaching

And What Is Your Fee?

How much do you charge? What is your fee?

How many times have you asked that question? How many times have you been asked that question?

As a person that is self-employed or running your own business, how do you feel when asked that question? What goes through your mind, and how do you respond?

It is true that one must be reasonable, both the person who charges and the person who is paying for the services. You need to consider your training, time, money, and energy you have invested in your pursued occupation. How good are you at what you are doing? Is it your passion? How much is it worth? How much do you value what you are doing?

A spouse sent her husband (a shop owner) over to me for a hypnotherapy session. She wanted to discover why it was that they never had enough money. Although work was abundant, he had lots of clients and good employees, his business did not generate enough money to even support his own family.

During the hypnotherapy session, he revealed that many customers would drop in at his shop unannounced with a small job that would only take him just 5 minutes to fix. He explained he did not fee justified to charge for something so simple. By making him aware of the total time taken each day by "Small-Job-Drop-Ins", he realized his productivity was down 50 percent…and so was his income.

I asked him to consider the number of years he spent in trade school and then to add the number of years he was an apprentice and a journeyman. The total, I recall, was 17 years. When I asked how well and how fast he thought that "a small job" would be done by an unskilled tradesman, my client was speechless.

Your Notes

Anny's Teaching

Deepening his trance, I then suggested that, in reality, the "five minutes jobs" were actually the results of 17 years of experience + five minutes of expertise and charging an appropriate and reasonable fee for services rendered was justified. This shift in the worth of his expertise improved his life.

I experienced this for myself recently. I called a service man to repair my overhead garage door which would not open properly and made worrisome noises as I struggled to have it close.

The repair man pushed the open/close button a few times, went to his van and came back with a step ladder, a hammer, and a screwdriver. He went up the stepladder, unscrewed something, gave one rail a good blow with the hammer, screwed the thing back on, got down the stepladder, and it was done! It took him about 15 minutes total and then he handed me the bill. The charge was for one hour.

As I was happily writing him a cheque for the amount requested, the service man, (genuinely puzzled by my behaviour) mentioned that I looked happy.

Of course I was, I said! He had been working for the company during the summer vacations for four years, went to NAIT for apprenticeship in that field for two years (if my memory serves me well) and was working full time as a tradesman for three years now.

I explained that, had he not known what he was doing, the repair could have cost me much more than the one hour he charged. In my view, I was paying that amount for 4+2+3 =9 years and 15 minutes. I truly believed I had received great value for the money I paid.

Our hidden ideas about self-worth and the worth of certain skills lead me to explore and then incorporate some important questions/training during class with the hypnotherapy students. As I lead the class to experience a mini regression at the beginning of the training as hypnotherapist I lead the class into a hypnotized mini regression where I say: "As you take a

Your Notes

Anny's Teaching

deep breath, and exhale, allow your mind to slide back to something that impressed your mind on how a healer should be paid, ...just go there...find yourself there..." The answers inevitably reveal how well each student is going to do for themselves as self-employed Hypnotherapist – not based on how good they are at it but solely based on the past belief they have! However, I then follow this up with a journey back within to address their beliefs in a way that will be more beneficial to them.

It is also important to investigate what you think about your field of occupation. What is your belief about what and how a person should be paid in your field of occupation? Deep down inside, do you respect that field of occupation? How do you expect to do well and to be successful? How do you expect to be paid? The answers to these questions will ultimately always reveal why someone is not making a good living in the field of their choice.

Other valid questions to ask yourself are: What are my beliefs regarding money, and where do these beliefs come from? If your belief is "Money is the root of all evil" how do you want to have an abundance of money with this kind of belief?

On the other hand, how much do you value the goods or the service rendered?

Also, do you need something that will do or do you want something that will last – that has both quality and quantity?

There was a "special buy" sale on six-volt batteries. We needed one, so we bought two at that price. As usual, my husband wrote the date put into service on top of the "radar light" battery. It went dead very quickly compared to the ones we usually buy. How come? The dismantled six volt "radar light" batteries revealed 16 batteries in the regular one compared to only 12 batteries in the "Special Buy" one.

Your Notes

Anny's Teaching

This reminds me of a regular hypnotherapy client that came to me over a period of a few years, driving about three hours one way for her hypnotherapy session. Then for a stretch of time, I did not see her.

When she came back to me she said:

"Anny, there is a new hypnotherapist in my town and I did not have to drive that far to see her. She also cost less. So I changed over to her. But after two years of regular therapy sessions with her, I have not seen any progress with myself or my issues. It was a waste of time and money. I should have stayed with you. Although you may cost more by the hour, you greatly benefit me much more.

So when you ask "how much?", is your focus on cost, or is your focus on value?

The choice is yours. So is the outcome.

Anny

Your Notes

Anny's Teaching

What Do You See?

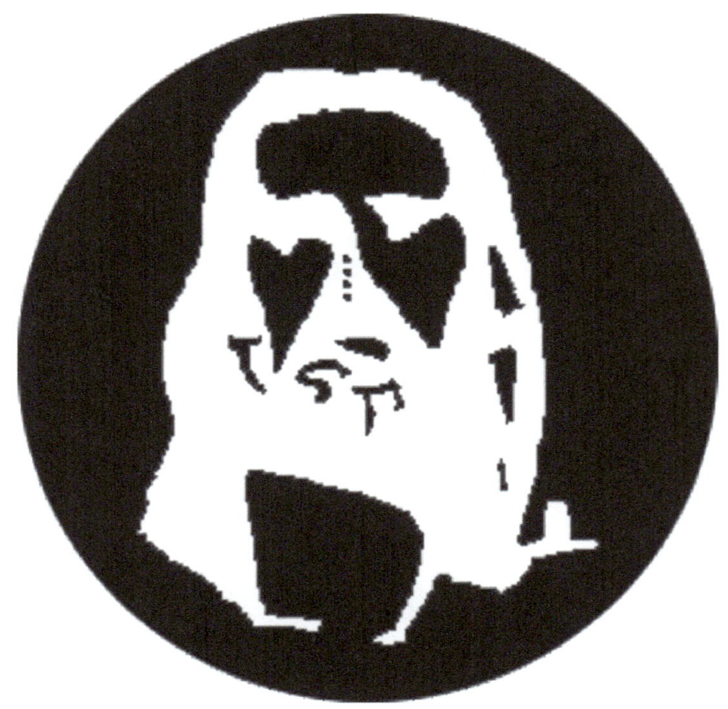

What do you see?

Concentrate on the four black dots for 30 seconds.

Close your eyes and tilt your head back.

You will see a white circle, keep focused on the circle.

What do you see?

Your Notes

Anny's Teaching

The Original No Suggestion Suggestion

By Drake Eastburn received during Anny's Hypno-Fertility training in Toronto, Ontario, Canada in July 2009.

This is an adaptation to Milton Erickson end of sessions as printed in HYP 201, the red book.

I wonder how much you remember what I said seven minutes before (chose any length of time when applicable)

and your conscious mind can remember to forget or forget to remember whatever I said, the choice is yours.

And your subconscious mind will remember this and work in it, and it will be so.

When giving this suggestion, I add *much to your surprise and delight.*

You can adapt your own way at giving this suggestion. I like the idea and use a variation of this no suggestion suggestion. It is fun and works very well.

Anny

Your Notes

Anny's Teaching

Please note: In this document, the word changes in the original document are shown here in italic as *improvements.*

At some point I am going to be giving you a suggestion, a very special, a very powerful suggestion, so powerful in fact that this suggestion is effective one hundred percent of the time.

Very few people have ever received this very special, very powerful suggestion.

However, because of some of the things that you said during the interview process, I now know that you are ready, willing, and able to receive this suggestion, fully and completely, body, mind, and spirit.

NOW, there is a side effect to this suggestion, and that side effect is that you will not remember this suggestion. It does not matter that you will not remember this suggestion, because I am going to slip in this suggestion in such a way that you will not even notice it.

It does not matter that you will not remember this suggestion because your subconscious mind knows the suggestion. Yes, your subconscious mind knows this suggestion and your subconscious mind enjoys this suggestion.

And because your subconscious mind enjoys this suggestion, your subconscious mind embraces this suggestion. Because your subconscious mind embraces this suggestion, good, healthy positive *improvements* occur, in your life, not the least of which is … … … …

(insert***): client's specifics such as you have greater confidence***

all because of this one very special, very powerful suggestion that I am going to give you at some point, that you will not even remember.

Your Notes

Anny's Teaching

Now, other good, healthy, positive *improvements* will occur as well, all because of this one very special, very powerful suggestion and something I refer to as the domino effect.

Yes, any time we take control in our lives just as you are doing right this very moment by … … … …

(insert client's specifics here, or say nothing at all),

it is as if you are knocking over that first domino and the rest of the dominos begin to topple and other good, healthy, positive *improvements* begin to fall right into your life.

Some of these good, healthy, positive *improvements* will be fairly obvious like … … … …

(client specific or not).

You have a great deal more energy. You feel like doing more vigorous, more active kinds of things and you do more vigorous, more active kinds of things.

You think more clearly. You have a new, more positive attitude, a new optimism; you are always looking ahead to each new day, knowing that good things are coming your way. You blaze the trail for others to follow. Yes, you set the example that others follow.

Now, other good healthy, positive *improvements* will occur as well, *improvements* might be, I can only be speculating and most likely so would you.

However, it is nice to know that the subconscious mind knows exactly which good, healthy, positive *improvements* you are up for and in what order they need to occur. It is nice to know that consciously there is not much you need to think about. There is not much you need to do. It is nice to know that the subconscious mind just takes care of everything.

Your Notes

Anny's Teaching

Now, some of these *improvements* may occur on a fairly subtle level. And you may be someone who is aware on a subtle level, or perhaps the hypnosis helps you to be more aware on a subtle level; it really does not matter at all.

As you may know, sometimes things that occur on SUBTLE LEVEL HAVE A VERY PROFOUND EFFECT UPON US – BODY, MIND AND SPIRIT. All because of this one very special, very powerful suggestion and the domino effect.

END.

Your Notes

Anny's Teaching

"The Building" Regression Technique

A regression technique I developed in the fall of 2007.

It was the third time my client was coming, with no improvement at all. He was stubborn and all in his head. He had a solid mental block nicely hidden, holding on to the benefit of doing so.

Then, out of the blues I "winged" this technique, having decided that that mental block will show itself, crystal clear. And it did.

A useful regression technique to use when a client cannot "unhook" a belief or situation, or when a client is all in their head: The Analyzer!

So far and to my knowledge, this is the best technique to make the client realize the "trigger that makes them fall back in a particular behavior.

Glossary

Important: Allow the client to figure this out as they go through the session.

A very beautiful and tall building – A kind of skyscraper

The representation of client's life as it is to be intended.

Each floor number

The client's life at the age of the floor number.

Your Notes

Anny's Teaching

Basement floors

B - 1, fetus – from 8 weeks gestation to birth
B - 2, embryo – from conception to 8 weeks gestation
B - 3, past life

Elevator

The client's subconscious mind

Please note: *It was suggested a client would know how long they will live by knowing the number of floors in the building they are in. After much soul searching, I have decided to stay out of mentioning the building total height, since sometimes I make my client go 10, 20 or more years ahead to look back to now and realize how they will (most likely) look at the present situation they perceive they are in now.*

Basic Instructions

After leading a client into a trance, make them contemplate their reason they decided to come for therapy.

As they are contemplating what they came for, make them find themselves in front of a very beautiful and tall building. A kind of skyscraper. Tall, slender, and beautiful.

As they are entering the building, ask your client to walk to the elevator. A double door elevator.

Observing their surroundings, make your client realize this building is a representation of their life.

Finding themselves in front of the elevator, explain to the client that this elevator functions on automatic. There is only one little window showing

Your Notes

Anny's Teaching

one digital set of number indicating where the elevator is at the present time.

A number shows the elevator is at the present time on the ________ floor *(The floor number is their present age number).*

Standing in front of the elevator, contemplating what they came for, wondering where and when did it start, the floor indicator shows the elevator is coming down, down, down *(use this as a deepening technique).*

A bell rings gently, indicating the elevator has arrived.

The doors open, and suggest to the client to step into the elevator, a very beautiful elevator. Something they never could imagine an elevator could be so beautiful and comfortable.

As they are there, truly enjoying this wonderful elevator, the doors close and the elevator functioning on full automatic starts to gently move **as you make your client contemplate what they came for, wondering what is it all about, where and when did it start**.

Ask your client to let you know when the elevator stops, and at which floor.

What is interesting is that the elevator will stop at the decision point, when the mind was impressed by the idea.

As the doors open, ask the client to step out on that floor, and meet themselves at the age indicated by the floor number.

Regular routine: *Say hi, give them a hug, walk through their life at that age, and re-visit that age.*

Suggest to your client to find a place where they can talk in total privacy with the younger one and ask how are things, what is going on, and what

Your Notes

Anny's Teaching

does that have to do with what they came for, wondering where and when did it start.

Should the younger one not know what happened or not admit it started at that age, ask if they would like to find out more. Together with the younger self, ask client to stand in from of the elevator, the doors open, step into the elevator and as they are both contemplating what they came for, wondering where and when did it start, the doors will close, and the elevator will start moving again.

Please note: *If the issue started at the age indicated by the floor number, the elevator doors will close as they are making themselves comfortable and stay at that floor, not moving or sometimes the elevator doors will simply stay open!*

To make sure the elevator (the subconscious mind) will indicate the age the issue started, let the client find out by themselves that each floor is an age.

Also, only tell client where they are if they find themselves in the basement: Floor B- 1 – fetus, Floor B- 2 - embryo, Floor B-3 - past life.

Towards the end of the session ask the client to update the younger self/selves by going to the floor of the client's present age.

End by going down to the first floor, either taking the younger self/selves with them or dropping them off at their own floor.

Wrap the session up as usual

Note: *I found out it works very well when the session is the third one or more. I use it when it becomes obvious to get the information out of the client's subconscious will be like pulling teeth. My clients are elated each time ... "because there was no struggle at all" as one stated.*

This method works so well I used it a few times at the first session with very analytical clients. Well, to my chagrin, it did not work at all.

Your Notes

Anny's Teaching

ISBN 0-19-500223-7

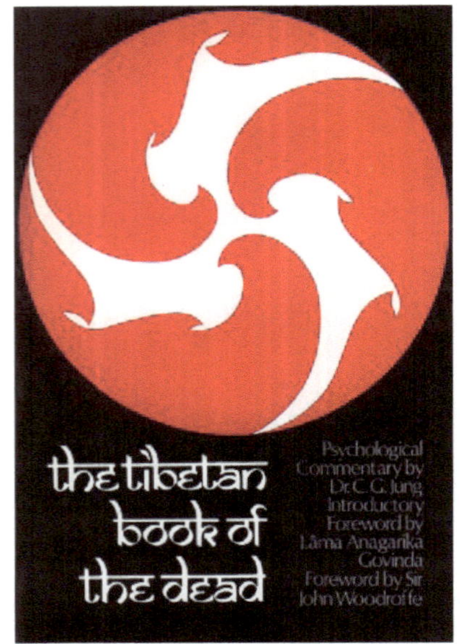

The Tibetan Book Of The Dead

First published in 1927, The Tibetan Book of the Dead, or the Bardo Thödol, has since been revised and reprinted in several editions; for the Galaxy Books edition, Dr. Evans-Wentz prepared a special preface.

Although the Bardo Thödol is used in Tibet as a breviary, and read or recited on the occasion of death, it was originally conceived to serve as a guide not only for the dying and the dead, but for the living as well. As a contribution to the science of death and of existence after death, and of rebirth, The Tibetan Book of the Dead is unique among the sacred books of the world.

"Dr. Evans-Wentz, who literally sat at the feet of a Tibetan lama for years in order to acquire his wisdom … not only displays a deeply sympathetic interest in those esoteric doctrines, so characteristic of the genius of the East, but likewise possesses the rare faculty of making them more or less intelligible to the layman."

-Anthropology

The late W.Y. Evans-Wentz, formerly of Jesus College, Osford, is also the editor of The Tibetan Book of the Great Liberation (GB260), Tibet's Great Yogi, Milarepa (GB294), and Tibetan Yoga and Secret Doctrines (GB212)

Your Notes

Anny's Teaching

The Tibetan Book Of The Dead, Or The Bardo Thödol

Part 1: A Way Of Life

As you have observed **"A way of life",** the first part of this document please write down your impressions, what you have learned and your questions by watching this film.

Your Notes

Anny's Teaching

The Tibetan Book Of The Dead, Or The Bardo Thödol

Part 2: The Great Liberation

After having viewed the first part of this documentary about religion, as you have observed, "The Great Liberation", the second part of this documentary, The Tibetan Book of the Dead,

Please write down your impressions and what you have learned by watching this film.

This will facilitate a discussion about the questions of religions, beliefs, life and death.

Bardo Thödol,

Tibetan:

"Liberation in the Intermediate State Through Hearing"
also called Tibetan Book of the Dead.

In Tibetan Buddhism, a funerary text that is recited to ease the consciousness of a recently deceased person through death and assist it into a favorable rebirth.

Your Notes

Anny's Teaching

Other Lives, Other Selves

A Jungian Psychotherapist Discovers Past Lives.

Made at a workshop to therapists, this film illustrated the remarkable power of past life regression. Featuring the work of Dr. Roger Woolger, a certified Jungian analyst. It shows how past lives are a springboard for understanding our current problems.

While not discounting the possibility that these past lives stories could all be fantasies, Dr. Woolger feels that "If the unconscious mind believes them, it does not matter whether they are true or not."

Woolger looks at the way the person is reliving this story in his or her current own current life. This is where past life *regressio*n becomes present life *therapy*.

By stressing forgiveness, positive affirmation and learning to die, the chronic pain and illness in these past life injuries is astonishingly eradicated.

He explains, for example, how someone abandoned by his parents and left to die in a past life would be afraid of relationships in the current life.

To facilitate a review or what may be called debriefing, please write down your questions as you are watching this film as well as when you are pondering about what you have observed.

Your Notes

Anny's Teaching

Chakras

The Sanskrit word Chakra literally translates to wheel or disk.

In yoga, meditation, and Ayurveda, this term refers to wheels of energy throughout the body. There are seven main chakras, which align the spine, starting from the base of the spine through to the crown of the head.

To visualize a chakra in the body, imagine a swirling wheel of energy where matter and consciousness meet.

This invisible energy, called Prana, is vital life force, which keeps us vibrant, healthy, and alive.

Source: The Chopra Center

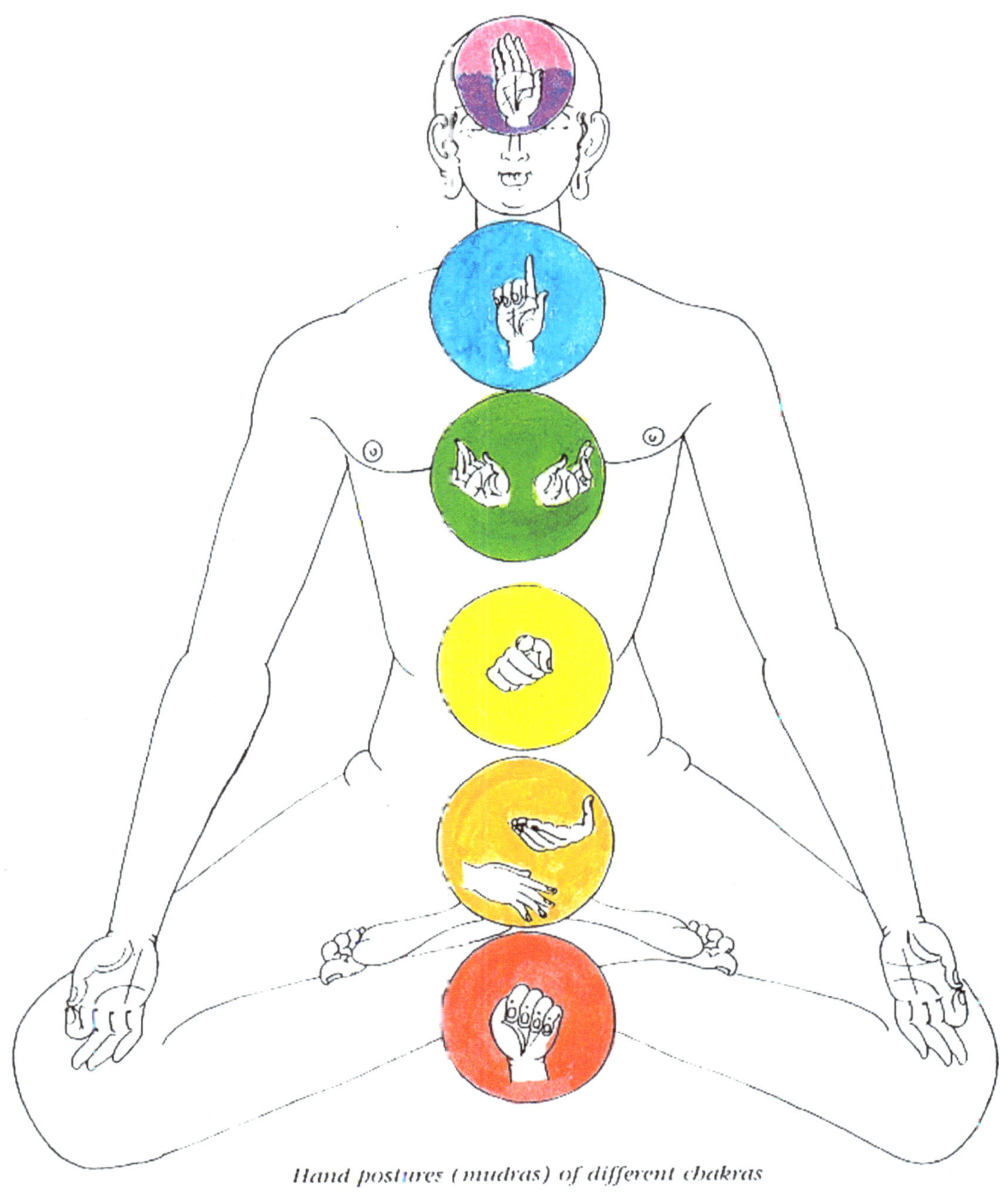

Hand postures (mudras) of different chakras

Source: Chakras, Energy Centers of Transformation, by Harish Johari

Body Language

The body is reflecting what is going on at soul level.

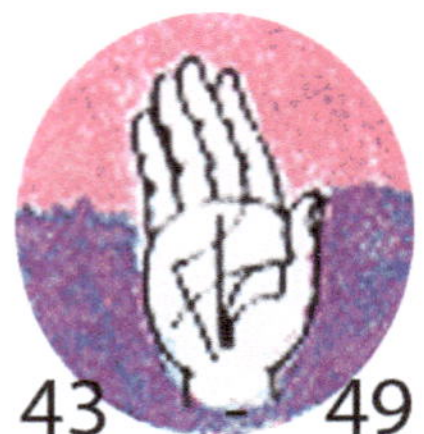

Integrating with the source. An understanding beyond comprehension. We actively attempt to integrate ourselves with the understanding of God - to bring our exterior and interior lives together into a harmonious whole with the source.

A tendency of having things done for us. *That goes on for the rest of our lives.*

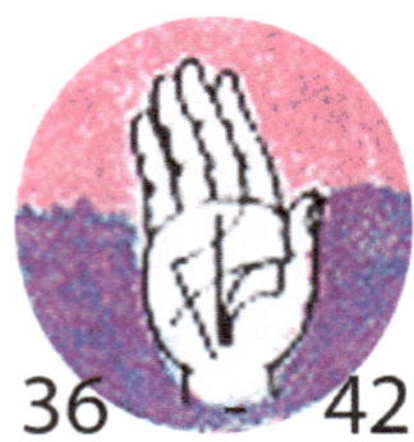

Second step of what we will do next. The lifestyle, the wisdom & spiritual age. Less fear. Start to see clearly for our self and other people's lives. We begin seriously to question our spiritual nature as it relates to the lifestyle we have created. All the knowledge we have gained begins to transmute to a kind of wisdom.

At this point, we decide to develop our spiritual nature or we affirm the consequences of avoiding this growth.

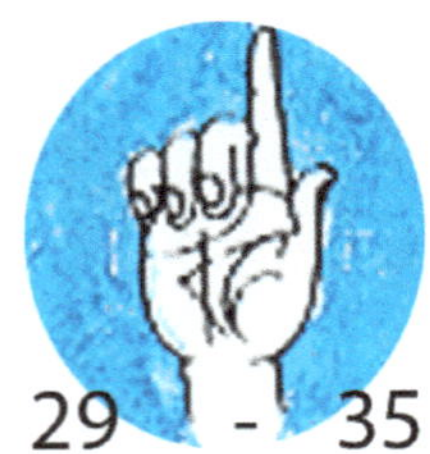

First step of what we will do next. Re-evaluation, drinking, affairs, job changing. Want to create the better world to be in.

This is the time when we become profoundly aware that

how we express ourselves is how we live with others.

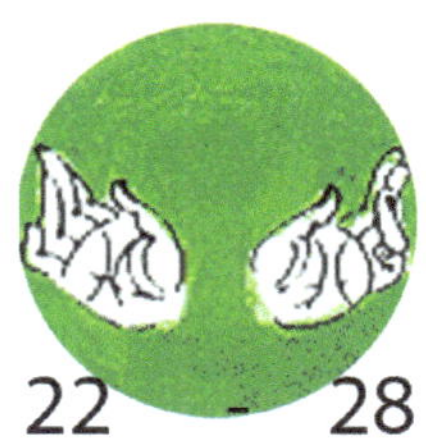

We want more harmony. Compassion, understanding, love. Human relation to love, self-love, mature love. Stuck into the drama, the security and be noticed. We start to develop our relationship to love - self-love and mature love of others - and abilities of evaluation and decision in terms of lifestyle.

At this point, we decide how harmonious we desire to be in life.

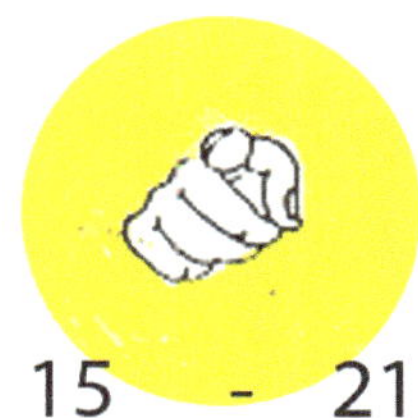

Emotional issues. Sense of right. Control, prestige. Wanting power, throwing their weight around, the top dog.

We deal with issues of emotionality relating to other people, the assessment of personal power, and the practice of free will: all the problems of adolescence are felt here.

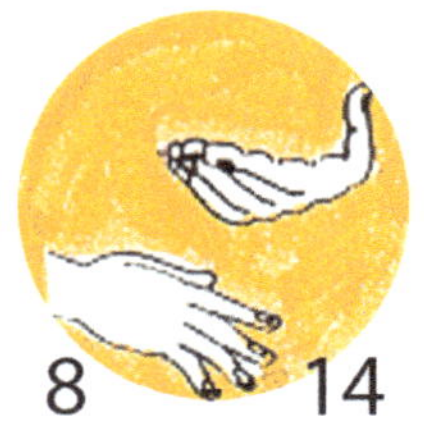

Sensation. Desiring money, sex, God or anything else. Cannot differentiate others from ours - emotionally.

Our sexuality develops and produces crises of various kinds so that the human being can develop the subjective mind, the capacity for creativity and for fuller consciousness of self-identity.

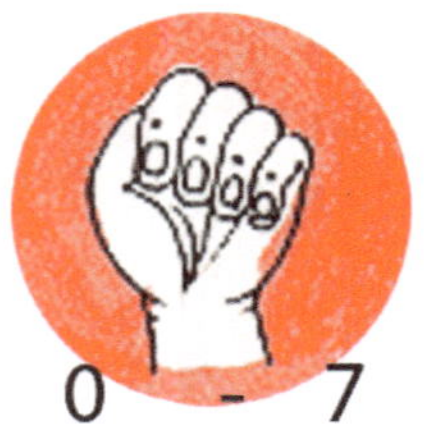

Security. Hording things. I want stuff. Grabbing. Petrified to make changes. Feeling stuck, lack of self-confidence, very moody, suicidal. At this point, our life revolves around survival and instincts of adjusting to the physical earth-plane experience.

One learns to crawl, walk, run, eat, and accept the physical expression of embracing, being loved and caressed, and so on. We develop our sense of balance until the physical form securely anchors itself to the Earth, according to how effectively the emotional experiences occur, and then prepares for its process of assimilating, of learning.

Source: Chakra workshop with Monica Tremblay and Going Within, by Shirley McLaine

The Body Is Reflecting What Is Going On "Inside"

The Body is Reflecting What is Going on "Inside"

Source: The Palmistry Workbook, by Nathaniel Altman

SPATULATED FINGER

Energetic, active, realistic, impulsive, down-to-earth, self-confident.

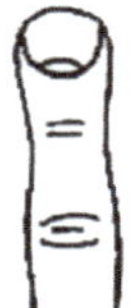

SQUARE FINGER

Loves order and regularity, perseverance, foresight, structured rational decisive action

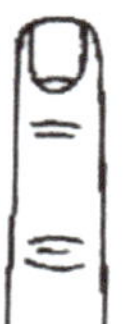

CONIC FINGER

Artistic, receptive to outer stimuli, sensitive, restless impulsive, institntual.

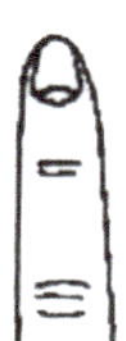

PSYCHIC FINGER

Strongly affected by outside stimuli, sensitive dreamy, intuitive, mediumistic.

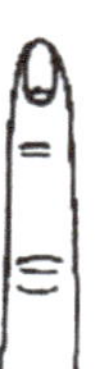

ROUND FINGER

Adaptable, well-rounded, balanced, active yet receptive, mental yet emotional.

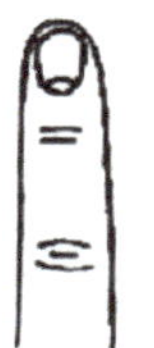

FLAT THUMB

Tendency to be highly strung and nervous

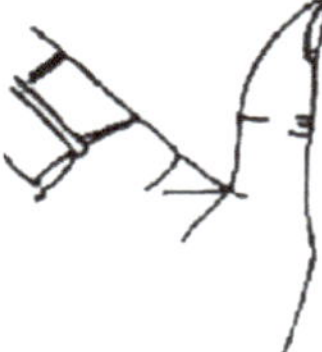

MURDERER'S THUMB

Tends to withhold energy to such an extent that strong, sudden bursts of temper can result.

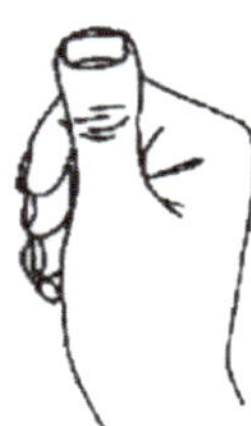

WAISTED THUMB

When the logic phalange is "waisted" logic is not a major aspect of the personality.

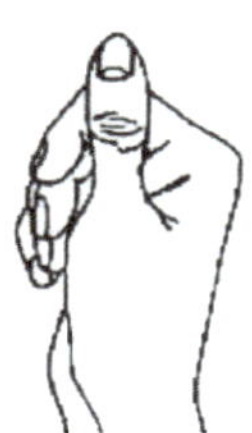

SUPPLE THUMB

Indicates emotional versatility and an ease to adapt. Too flexible: poor willpower.

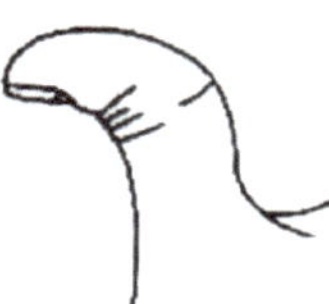

STIFF THUMB

Stubborn, prudent, tremendous difficulty adapting to new ideas and situations.

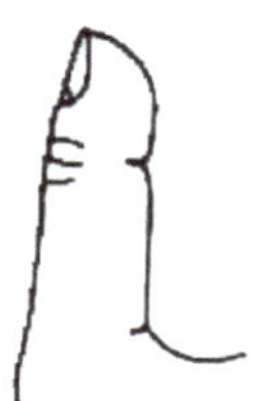

Source: The Palmistry Workbook, by Nathaniel Altman and Anny Slegten

Fingernails are like an open book: they reveal the physical condition of a person, the result of "what is going on inside". For example, white spots indicate inadequate nutrition and/or enemia; blue nails, poor blood circulation. Soft nails often indicate protein and calcium deficiency while brittle and broken nails can be a sign of an underactive thyroid or pituitary gland.

Here are a few examples of shapes, lines, and ridges.

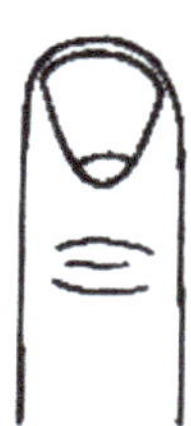

FAN-SHAPED NAILS AND LONG, NARROW NAILS

May indicate nervous disorders and psychosomatic diseases. It may also indicate fear and low tolerance for frustration.

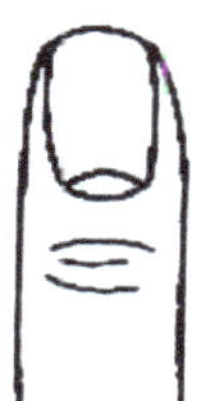

SHORT NAIL

Highly critical and impatient towards themselves, others and life. Prone to heart trouble and depression.

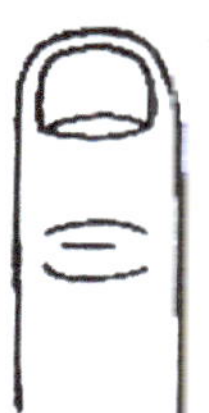

"WATCHGLASS" NAIL

Holding one's breath, not breathing. General weakness of the respiratory system.

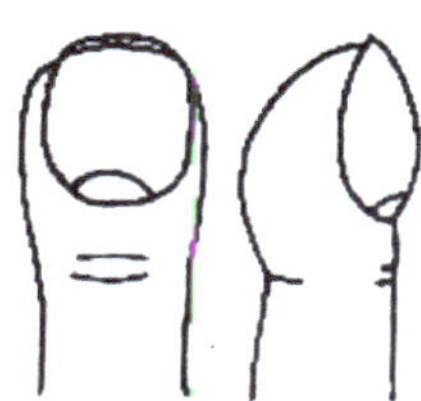

SPOON NAIL

Iron deficiency and underactive thyroid gland. Constant fatigue and lethargy. Poor sexual performance.

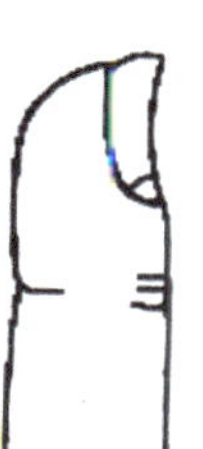

BEAU'S LINE OR DENT(S)

Severe emotional shock. Takes six months to move upwards as the nail grows. Results of the shock may physically appear when line reaches top of nail.

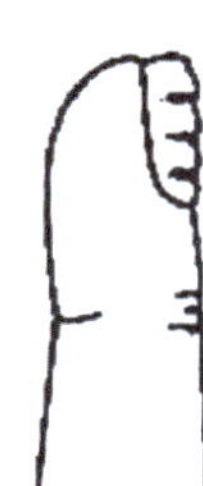

MEE'S LINES

High fever, arsenic poisoning, and coronary heart disease.

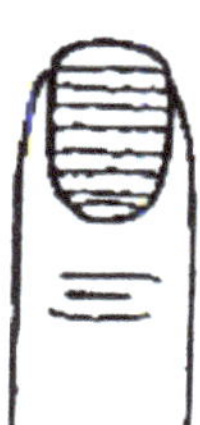

LONGITUDINAL RIDGES

Constant stress. Usually on thumb nails only. When finger nails too, indicates extreme stress.

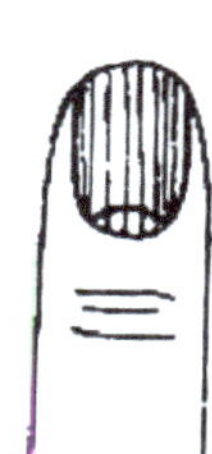

Eye Accessing Cues

While most people lump all of their internal information processing together and call it "thinking", Bandler and Grinder have noted that it can be very useful to divide thinking into the different sensory modalities in which it occurs. When we process information internally, we can do it visually, auditorily, kinesthetically, olfactorily, or gustatorily. As you read the word "circus", you may know what it means by seeing images of circus rings, elephants, or trapeze artists; by hearing carnival music; by feeling excited; or by smelling and tasting popcorn or cotton candy. It is possible to access the meaning of a word in any one, or any combination, of the five sensory channels.

Bandler and Grinder have observed that people move their eyes in systematic directions, depending upon the kind of thinking they are doing. These movements are called eye accessing cues. The chart indicates the kind of processing most people do when moving their eyes in a particular direction. A small percentage of individuals are "reversed", that is, they move their eyes in a mirror image of this chart. Eye accessing cues are discussed in chapter I of *Frogs into Princes*, and an in-depth discussion of how this information can be used appears in *Neuro-Linguistic Programming, Volume I*.

This chart on the following page is easiest to use if you simply superimpose it over someone's face, so that as you see them looking in a particular direction, you can also visualize the label for that eye accessing cue.

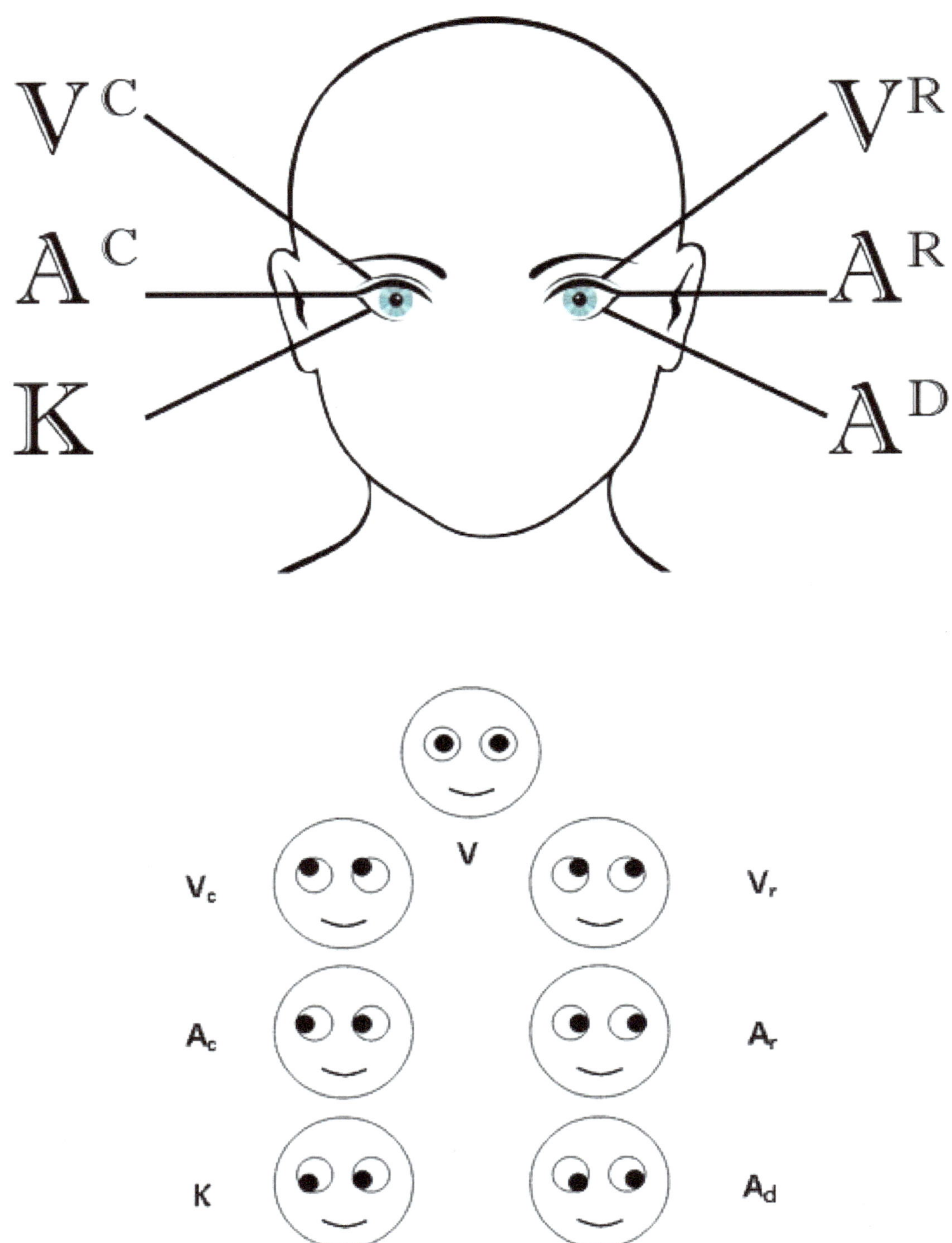
V C
A C
K
V R
A R
A D
V
V c
V r
A c
A r
K
A d

V^r ***Visual remembered:***
Seeing images of things seen before, in the way they were seen before. Sample questions that usually elicit this kind of processing include, "What color are your mother's eyes?" or "What does your coat look like?"

V^c ***Visual constructed:***
Seeing images of things never seen before, or seeing things differently than they were seen before. Questions that usually elicit this kind of processing include, "What would an orange hippopotamus with purple spots look like?" or "What would you look like from the other side of the room?"

A^r ***Auditory remembered:***
Remembering sounds heard before. Questions that usually elicit this kind of processing include, "What's the last thing I said?" or "What does your alarm clock sound like?"

A^c ***Auditory Constructed:***
Hearing sounds not heard before. Questions that tend to elicit this kind of processing include, "What would the sound of clapping turning into the sound of birds singing sound like?" or "What would your name sound like backwards?"

A^d ***Auditory digital:***
Talking to oneself. Questions that tend to elicit this kind of processing include, "Say something to yourself that you often say to yourself" or "Recite the Pledge of Allegiance".

K ***Kinesthetic:***
Feeling emotions, tactile sensations (sense of touch), or proprioceptive feelings (feelings of muscle movement). Questions to elicit this kind of processing include: "What does it feel like to be happy?" or "What is the
feeling of touching a pine cone?" or "What does it feel like to run?"

Put It On The Shelf

There is more to it when looking straight up, the reason I am enclosing this article:

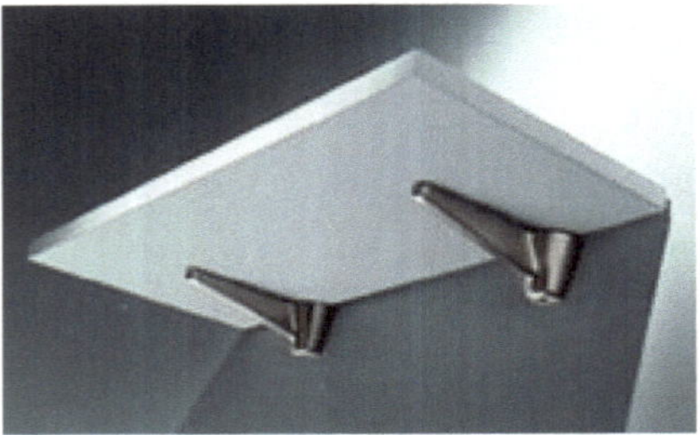

The joy of teaching and being in this profession is that students share their awareness with me. As you know, on the first day of class, I explain that sometimes what is taught challenges their beliefs.

Gesturing, I then ask when that happens, to please put whatever they do not agree with on the shelf for future assessment. It is with the student's permission and with gratitude that I am sharing with you a letter I just received:

Subject: "Put it on the shelf"

I had a realization of why the "put it on the shelf" visualization works so effectively. I want to share it with you.

I found myself contemplating the circumstances leading to an event. After achieving some progress, I began to notice a deep sadness within me. Understanding that I had reached a point that I was no longer making progress and just sitting in the feeling of sadness, I decided to "put it on the shelf", sleep on it, and come back to it.

I noticed the picture in my mind of this decision. I reached into my chest, pulled the feeling of sadness out of my chest, and placed it up onto the shelf above my head. As it moved upward from my chest to the shelf I felt the feeling of sadness dissipate completely.

This brought my thoughts to something you had mentioned in class. When someone looks up, they are avoiding emotion. When they look down, they are accessing the emotion. This is the reason we bring their focus down (for example, into their chest) to bring them into their emotion.

I then realized the true power of the shelf analogy.

When someone is uncomfortable or unsure of their feelings, belief, or attitude about what they are being told, putting that "up" on the shelf moves it to a place out of emotion. There it can sit on the shelf, objectively without judgement of good or bad, right or wrong, for as long as it wants to, without hitting the "save button".

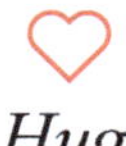

Hugs

Eye Movement Desensitization Reprocessing

EMDR Therapy Proves Rapid Eye Movement Eases Trauma

(source unknown, author Jillian Millar)

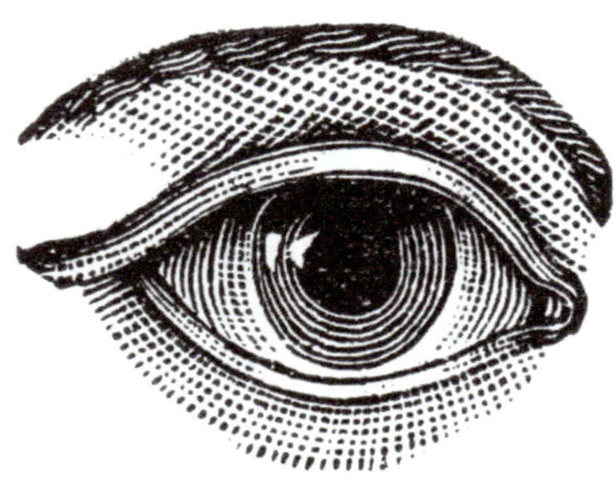

Ever thought the eyes are the window to the soul? A treatment involving eye movement may help us get past our most painful memories.

Trauma victims are discovering that EMDR (Eye Movement Desensitization Reprocessing) therapy allows them to work through the emotions associated with a crisis and recover more quickly.

Sheldon Walker, a Calgary therapist, has been offering the treatment for about three years. "When I went to take the training I was very skeptical. It was unlike the usual 'talking' therapy I do," he says.

When he began to use EMDR therapy in his practice, he was pleasantly surprised. "It was astounding because you could see that when people talked about painful issues their shoulders would lift, their whole demeanor would change and mostly they started to forgive themselves."

EMDR therapy was discovered in 1989 when California clinical psychologist Dr. Francine Shapiro discovered the treatment spontaneously.

Shapiro a cancer survivor, noticed that some of the painful emotions associated with her illness lost some of their sting after rapid eye movement.

She went on to test her theory, particularly with those suffering from Post-Vietnam Syndrome. Her patients followed her hand with their eyes as she asked them about their painful memories. Many found that the therapy calmed the emotions around the recollection.

Walker says that although no one knows exactly why EMDR therapy works, Shapiro has speculated that the process may replicate the inner work done during REM sleep. “It is thought that when a person has an unpleasant experience, dreaming is supposed to file it somewhere acceptable in the unconscious," he says. "But when the experience is just too terrible, the issue does mot get resolved.

This is like a digestion process where you do rapid eye movement and that allows natural healing." "When you introduce rapid eye movement, like a dream, it does seem to reprocess painful memories and desensitize the pain and negative feelings that go with the memory.
The person does not lose the memory, but when they bring it forward the next time, it does not seem to have the punch it used to."
Walker says one of the most noticeable things about the therapy is that it decreases the sense of guilt associated with the incident. "It seems to resolve the belief that the person was to blame. It makes them realize that they were just a victim," says Walker.

"This has an effect on their whole life. If you grow up thinking you are bad, you are dirty and you need to be punished – and suddenly you do not think that anymore – it just changes a persons’ feelings about themselves on many levels."

Though Shapiro describes the process in detail in her book, Walker recommends that professional who want to offer the therapy should take the training available. "Often a client will present you with one memory or issue, and then there are a multitude of issues they bring."

Eye Movement Integration

Instructions To The Client

By Steven Andreas

The method you are about to experience is very simple.

First, I will ask you to think of a problem or limitation and notice how you experience it.

Then, *while you continue to think of this problem*, I will ask you to keep your head in one position as you smoothly follow the movement of the target in my hand with your eyes. You do not have to do anything else.

After following the target with your eyes for about 20 seconds, I will pause and ask you to tell me about any changes in how you experience the problem you are thinking of.

1. Most people will have an unpleasant feeling in response to thinking about the problem limitation. Using "100%" to rate the intensity of this feeling at the beginning, "80%" would mean that it *decreased* 20%; "120%" would mean that the intensity *increased* 20%. Or there might be no change.

2. There may also be qualitative changes.

   These could include:

   a. Perceptual changes in the way you think of the problem –for instance, your internal image could gain or lose color, or become smaller or larger, a voice or sound might increase or decrease in volume, or change in tone, etc.

b. Changes in the content of the problem – for instance, the person or event in the image might change, or the words that a voice says might change, etc.

c. Changes in the kind of feeling response to thinking about the problem – from fear to comfort, anger, or excitement, for instance.

d. Changes in the muscle tension or relaxation in all, or any part, of your body.

IMPORTANT

Please let me know what I can do to make this as comfortable and easy as possible for you. If you would like me to slow down or speed up, to hold the target farther away from your face or closer to you, to pause or stop at any time, or do more of a particular movement, or have any other suggestions, please let me know right away.

If at any time during this process you experience any discomfort, reluctance, or objections, please let me know immediately, so that we can stop and modify what we are doing.

Eye Movement Integration

Practitioner Worksheet

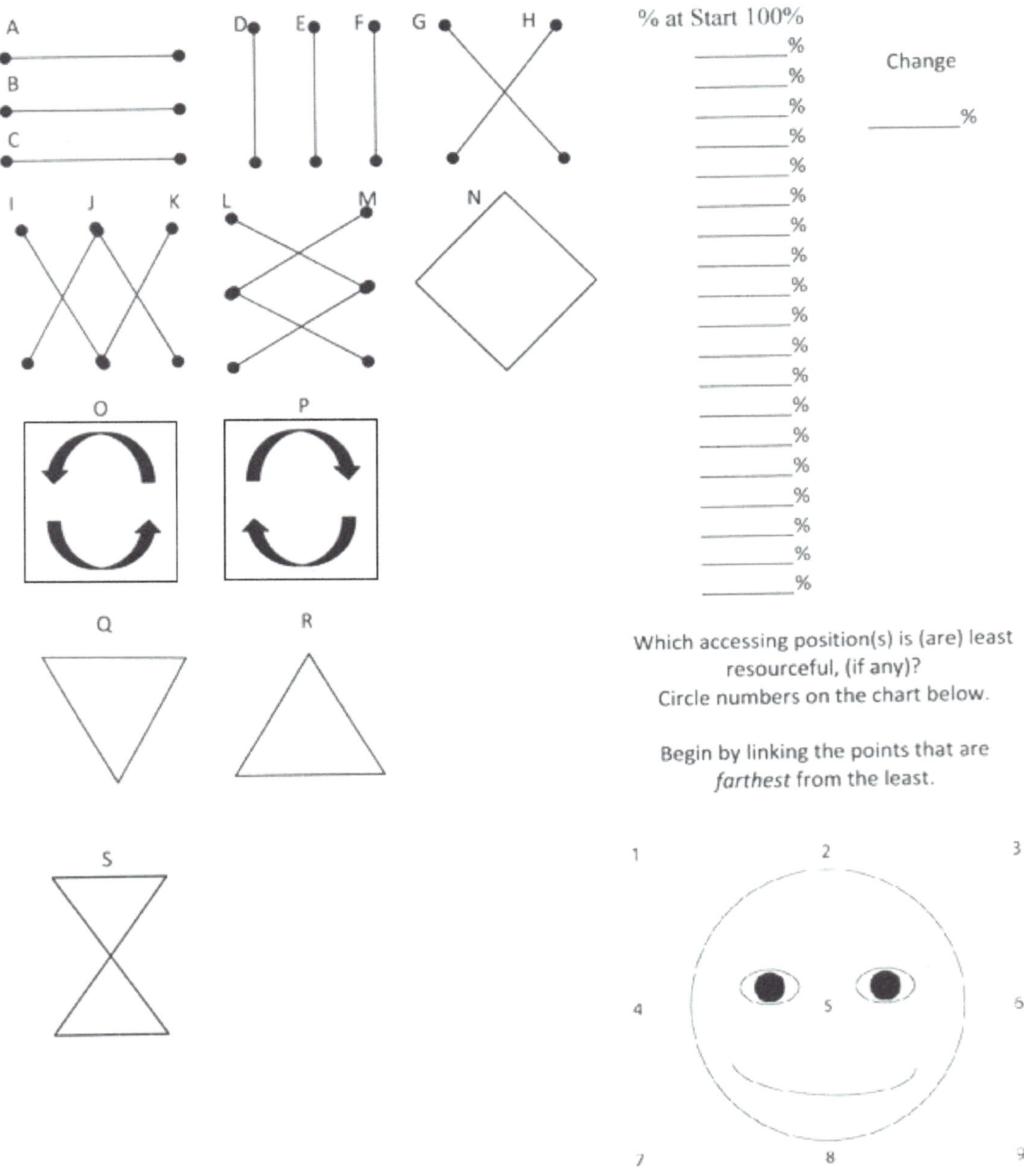

Client Worksheet

1. Briefly describe the kind of problem the client has chosen to work with: (unpleasant memory, present mood, headache or other physical symptom, anger, grief, etc.)

2. Predominant sub modalities of client's experience of this problem state:

Visual

____

____

Auditory

____

____

Kinesthetic

____

____

3. Which accessing position(s) is (are) least resourceful, (if any)?

(Circle numbers on the picture to the right.)

4. Begin by linking the points that are *farthest* from the least.

5. "Erase" any glitches that come up

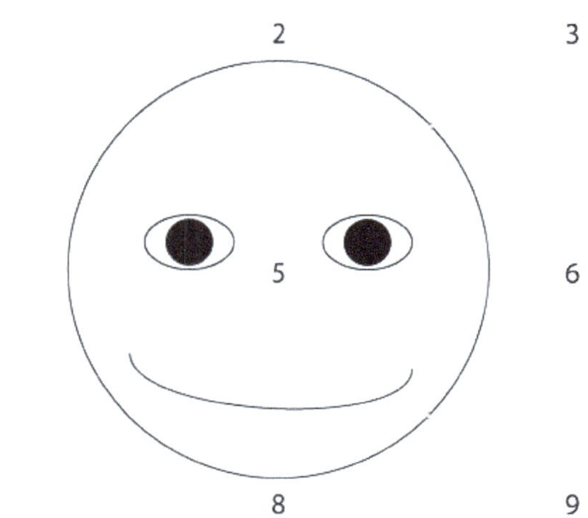

Questions You May Have About Hypnosis

1. EXACTLY WHAT IS HYPNOSIS?

Hypnosis is a state of altered consciousness that occurs normally in every person just before the person enters into the sleep state. In therapeutic hypnosis, we prolong this brief interlude so that we can work within its bounds.

2. CAN EVERYBODY BE HYPNOTIZED?

Yes, because it is a normal state that everybody passes through before going to sleep. However, it is possible to resist hypnosis like it is possible to resist going to sleep. But even if one resists hypnosis, with practice the resistance can be overcome.

3. WHAT IS THE VALUE OF HYPNOSIS?

There is no magic in hypnosis. There are some conditions in which it is useful and others in which no great benefit is derived. It is employed in medicine to reduce tension and pain which accompany various physical problems and to aid certain rehabilitative procedures. In psychiatric practice, it is helpful in short-term therapy, and also, in some cases, in long-term treatment where obstinate resistances have been encountered.

Your Notes

Anny's Teaching

4. WHO CAN DO HYPNOSIS?

Only a qualified professional person should decide whether one needs hypnosis or could benefit from it. The professional person requires special training in the techniques and uses of hypnosis before he can be considered qualified,

5. WHY DO SOME PEOPLE NOT BELIEVE IN THE VALUES OF HYPNOSIS?

Hypnosis is a much misunderstood phenomenon. The exaggerated claims made for it by undisciplined persons have turned some people into not feeling comfortable with it. Some doctors and psychiatrists too do not believe in the value of hypnosis, because Freud gave it up several decades ago, and because they themselves have not had too much experience with its modern uses.

6. CAN HYPNOSIS NOT BE SAFE?

The hypnotic state is as safe as the sleep state. Sometimes unskilled operators may give subjects foolish suggestions, such as one often witnessed in stage hypnosis, where the trance is exploited for entertainment purposes. A delicately balanced and sensitive person exposed to unwise and unkind suggestions may not respond favorably. On the whole, hypnosis is safe and comforting when practiced by ethical and qualified practitioners.

Your Notes

Anny's Teaching

7. DO I NEED HYPNOTHERAPY?

If you have nervous symptoms such as tensions, depression, fears, fatigue, and certain physical complaints for which your doctor finds no physical basis; if you find it difficult to get along at work or in your relations with people; if you have a school, sex or martial problem; or if you merely feel irritable, unhappy and believe you are not getting the most out of life, hypnotherapy will be of help to you.

8. HOW DOES HYPNOTHERAPY WORK?

Nervous symptoms and unwarranted unhappiness are the product of inner emotional conflicts. In hypnotherapy you are helped to understand your conflicts. In this way, it is possible for you to do something constructive about solving them.

9. CAN PHYSICAL SYMPTOMS BE CAUSED BY EMOTION?

Many physical symptoms are psychosomatic in nature, which means that they have an emotional or nervous basis. When you come to think of it, it is not really so strange that emotional strain or worry would produce physical symptoms. After all every organ in your body is connected with your brain by nerve channels; and so it is logical that when your nervous system is upset by some crisis or conflict, you may feel the effects in various organs of the body.

Your Notes

Anny's Teaching

10. IF I CANNOT SOLVE MY PERSONAL PROBLEMS WITHOUT HELP, DOES THAT MEAN THAT I HAVE A WEAK WILL OR AM ON THE WAY TO A MENTAL BREAKDOWN?

No. Even if you have no serious symptoms, it is difficult to work out emotional problems by yourself because you are too close to them and cannot see them clearly. More and more people, even those with a great deal of psychological knowledge are seeking help these days because they realize this. The fact that you desire aid is a compliment to your judgement and is no indication that you are not mentally stable. Hypnotherapy has helped countless numbers of people to overcome serious emotional symptoms, and has enabled many others to increase their working capacities and to better their relationships with people.

11. WHAT HAPPENS TO INFORMATION ABOUT ME?

In scientific work, records are necessary, since they permit of a more thorough dealing with one's problems. It is understandable that you might be concerned about what happens to the information about you, because much or all of this information is highly personal. Case records are confidential. No outsider, not even your closest friend or family physician is permitted to see your case record without your written permission.

Your Notes

Anny's Teaching

12. I AM NOT SURE I CAN BE HYPNOTIZED.

All people go through a state akin to hypnosis before falling asleep. There is no reason why you should not be able to enter a hypnotic state.

13. WHAT DOES IT FEEL LIKE TO BE HYPNOTIZED?

The answer to this is extremely important because it may determine whether or not you can benefit from hypnosis. Most people do not pursue hypnosis after a few sessions because they perceive that they are not suitable subjects. The average person has the idea that he will go through something different, new and spectacular in the hypnotic state. Often he equates being hypnotized with being anesthetized or being asleep or being unconscious. When in hypnosis he finds that his mind is active; that he is very aware of himself; and that he remembers everything that has happened when he opens his eyes. He believes himself to have not succeeded. He imagines then that he is not a good subject and he is apt to not continue hypnotic treatments. The experience of being hypnotized is the same as the experience of relaxing and of starting to go to sleep. Because this experience is so familiar to you, and because you may expect something startling different in hypnosis, you may not believe you are hypnotized when a trance is induced. Remember, you are conscious, you are fully aware. Your mind is active, your thoughts are under your control, you perceive all stimuli and you are in complete communication with the operator and yourself. The only unique thing you may experience is a feeling of heaviness in your arms, and tinglingness in your hands and fingers. If you are habitually a deep sleeper, you may doze momentarily or if you are a light sleeper, you may have a feeling you are completely awake.

Your Notes

Anny's Teaching

14. HOW DEEP DO I HAVE TO GO TO GET BENEFITS FROM HYPNOSIS?

If you can conceive of hypnosis as a spectrum of awareness that stretches from waking to sleep, you will realize that some aspects are close to the waking state, and share the phenomena of waking, and some aspects are close to sleep and participate in the phenomena of light sleep. But over the entire spectrum, suggestibility is increased and this is what makes hypnosis potentially beneficial provided we put the suggestibility to a constructive use. The depth of hypnosis does not always correlate with the degree of suggestibility. In other words, even if you go no deeper than the lightest stages of hypnosis and are merely mildly relaxed, you will still be able to benefit from its therapeutic effects. It so happens

that with practice, you should be able to go in deeper, but this really is not too important in the great majority of cases.

15. HOW DOES HYPNOSIS WORK?

The human mind is extremely suggestible and is being bombarded constantly with suggestive stimuli from and outside and suggestive thoughts and ideas from the inside. A good deal of suffering is the consequence of negative thoughts and impulses invading one's mind form conscious recesses. Unfortunately, past experiences, guilt feelings and repudiated impulses and desires are incessantly sabotaging one's happiness, health and efficiency. By the time one has reached adulthood, he has built up "negative" modes of thinking, they are not easy to break. In hypnosis, we attempt to replace these "negative" attitudes with "positive" one's. It takes time to disintegrate old habit patterns, so do not be discouraged if there is no immediate effect. If you continue to practice the principles taught you by your therapist, you will eventually notice change. Even though there may be no apparent alterations on the surface, a restructuring is going on underneath. An analogy may make this clear. If you hold a batch of white blotters above the level of your eyes so that

Your Notes

Anny's Teaching

you see the bottom blotter, you will observe nothing different for a while until sufficient ink has been poured to soak through the entire thickness. Eventually the ink will come down. During this period while nothing seemingly is happening, enough ink had been poured, we would be tempted to consider the process a failure. Suggestions in hypnosis are like ink poured on layers of resistance; one must keep repeating them before they come through to influence old, destructive patterns.

16. HOW CAN I HELP IN THE TREATMENT PROCESS?

It is important to mention to your therapist your reactions to treatment no matter how unfounded, unfair or unreasonable these reactions may seem. If for any reason you believe you should not continue the therapy, mention your desire to do so to your hypnotherapist. Important clues may be derived from your reactions, dreams and resistances that will provide an understanding of your inner conflicts, and help in your treatment.

17. WHAT ABOUT SELF-HYPNOSIS?

"Relaxing exercise", "self-hypnosis" and "auto-hypnosis" are interchangeable terms for a reinforcing process that may be valuable in helping your therapist help you. If this adjunct is necessary, it will be employed. The technique is simple and safe.

Questions About Gord's Session

- Question 1 -
- Question 2 -
- Question 3 -
- Question 4 -
- Question 5 -

Transcript: Asthma Attacks And Allergies

Please note: This is Gord's third session.

Gord: I am here because like you said I noticed changes. I am thinking positive but at the same time out of the blue a thought will just come and it will not be positive.

Anny: All what?

Gord: And I needed that. Without that. Without that on, right away I would get an asthma attack. And if I did that right away I would get an asthma attack. And if I just go like this, you get this tool and all that and right away I would be all stuffed up.

You know it would not take hardly anything. And other people are walking around all day without any protection but me just take one breath and I am – it is no good. And then one day I had my respirator on and, you know, and I was feeling good, no discomfort or anything, it was feeling really good, and I went back to the lunchroom and after lunch I thought oh I am going to see if I got rid of this or what the story is.

So I went out there without the respirator. I just stepped outside the lunch room and then I feel just a little bit oh, just a little bit and then I walk all the way to where I am supposed to be working and then it is really bad and then I have to walk all the way back and then I have to use the inhaler, get the respirator and every day was like that, every day.

So finally, I said to the foreman, look you have give me a layoff. It is no good for me down here.

Anny: But how many times do you work over there in that department?

Gord: When there is a really good job come up. This a gravy job. Everybody wants that job and you know it's 12 hour days and it's double time and well I could work there maybe three months a year. You know.

Anny: Gravy job, just before Christmas.

Gord: This time yah. Gravy job meaning money.

Anny: Oh I know that.

Gord: But it did not work for me.

Anny: You know, I wanted to mention something to you, but I thought I will not because. each time you mention something, you give it life. During the whole time you were fine, you always talked about it. I do not know if you noticed that. And I thought…

Gord: I talked about it.

Anny: Oh, yes. My asthma is gone..

Gord: I know. I know.

Anny: You kept saying that and I thought, we will see.

Gord: I know and try to twist my words around.

Anny: You were talking about allergies and asthma all the time.

Gord: Because I was so amazed it was gone. That was it, I was amazed.

Anny: Yes, but..

Gord: I would tell everybody.

Anny: Yes, but you were thinking about it.

Gord: Yah, of course.

Anny: So what do you expect?

Gord: I expect it is gone and it will stay gone.

Anny: No, the more you think lack of money, the more what is happening?

Gord: The more lack you have.

Anny: Well yah. And when you have a gravy job, you think about all the lack of money that is going to be gone.

Are you understanding something?

Gord: I do, I do, because I am listening to you, but I thought well. Because you know you have enough ideas in your head, I am keeping mine out.

Anny: Yes, and you kept telling me every morning you were thanking me to have taken the asthma away instead of saying you know it is so good to breathe easy. But no, you were talking about how it was before.

Gord: Okay, it feels good to breathe easy. Okay I could say that.

Anny: Yah, but that is not what you did.

Gord: No it is not what I did. It is just that simple.

Anny: You keep giving it life. You keep giving it life.

Gord: It is that simple. Okay I will have to change that.

Anny: Well, Yah, do not even talk about it. Just try to say, hey if you work with a pet, or a dog, or a cat or a donkey or whatever you were comparing to when you had asthma.

Gord: Yah, I thought it was gone and there would be no problem.

Anny: But the thing is, it was gone, but you then called it back.

Gord: I did hey? .

Anny: Well listen to what you kept saying. And I thought oh boy, well, we will see.

Gord: So I have to take that word out of my vocabulary all together?

Anny: Yes, yes. All stuffed up. And when you were feeling good, you would compare it to when you were all stuffed up and whatever.

Gord: So what do we do to fix it?

Anny: We will fix it. But take it out. Just like in the 101, I think I explained the boy with the bed wetting and then I said to the parents, I said no more, either he has a dry bed or he does not have a dry bed, and only talk about dry bed. And three months later he did not have a dry bed only once. That is all.

Gord: Yah, I forgot. I forgot about that.

Anny: So there are things you have to take out. I do not even think that I am breathing easily, because I do. I do not even think about it. Just like people who are overweight, all what they think about is what they can eat. Well. Hello, anybody home, what can you do if you think only about what you can eat? I do not even think about it. And when I open the fridge what do you feel, what do I feel like eating? And I eat it. And then Maurice you know has a sweet tooth. Then I am finished and so forth. And he gets in the curb all day. You should see it. And then he says do you want one? And I say no, I have enough, I have enough. I am full, that is it. It does not matter what you think.

Gord: That remind me of something too. A trigger to that thing I do not have.

Food. Food. If I eat some, and I thought oh, I will have a little bit more and I have a little bit more and I am full and I get congested. But I notice that. For any festivity, like Thanksgiving. The other day up in camp, it was Thanksgiving. A lot of nice turkey and ham and stuff and I had a big meal and stuffed up.

Anny: Well yah, you do not feel comfortable.

Gord: It is not just uncomfortable, it is just the way it goes. And I notice that quite a bit. And try to relate when does that happen the most. And that is one of them.

Anny: Is it not that interesting, when you do too much?

Gord: Yah, it stuffs me up. And the other time, when I am around sulfury sort of stuff.

Anny: A certain odour.

Gord: Yah, like the smell up in McMurray like is inside of an oil can. That sort of smell and sometimes there is sulfur and sometimes it just takes my breath away. And I was thinking last night, the wrong way of course. And I was in the bathroom and I am had a shower and I am so good, I am so good. As soon as I lay down in the bed, ah it is just a little bit.

Anny: And the thing is when you were up at camp and laying down, how was it?

Gord: It was too, it was a little bit. But by that time I already had a puff out of my inhaler, but it was not as bad as here.

Anny: Laying down at home huh.

Gord: Laying down in bed. Sitting up at the chesterfield, sometimes it got to me.

Anny: Yah, but from what you say is it is more at home than when you are somewhere else. Or more than when you are with someone in bed than when you are alone.

Gord: Not necessarily with someone. Just from the going upright to laying down. Just and I do not know I did not ever go into the living room to lay down to see what happened.

Anny: Yah to see if you got congested, right. Are you getting it?

Gord: See if I still feel well.

Anny: Yah, if you feel well there (pointing to his stomach).

Gord: Yah. Okay I get it.

Anny: See you are feeding it major. You are feeding it major, major, major.

Gord: Even when I am talking to you, I am trying to turn it around but I am not very successful at it.

Anny: You are making sure you do not let it go, do you not?

Gord: Yah, maybe I guess. Yah, but maybe just poor choice of words. If I had a better choice of words. Just like that. I just have to think a little bit more about what I say.

Anny: Gord, Gord, get it out of your vocabulary. But no, you are hanging onto it pretty good do you not? No way you are going to let go of that. And how is Suzy responding that you came home because of that?

Gord: I never told her I came home because of that. I told her I came home because of a layoff. But I did not want to open that can of worms at all.

Anny: Now I am going to ask you something. This is gravy work you went to huh? I do not want to know the numbers. But I would like to know the amount of money you made those days less the unexpected expenses, the total, compared to the same hours in another place.

Gord: I will tell you something else when I think about it. And normally, normally what you do is you look on the slip up top and it says the time you start work and when you start work, that is when they give you your orientation, your indoctrination, everything you have to know about your job to work safe.

But instead of doing it the normal way, they had that time up there, which was 7:30 at night, but they also had at the bottom, then it said report at 7:30 am to get your badge. So I go at 7:30 at night where they normally pick you up to start work and I phone for Jacob to come and get me and nobody came and nobody came and I waited all night.

And then finally I got ahold of someone that got ahold of someone else and she came over and said oh you were supposed to do that this morning. And I said no, no I am on night shift 7:30 pm. I even showed it to her. And said, why did they do that. So I lost a whole day right there and then I lost almost a $1,000 and so that is like….

Anny: And so okay, so you compare that to the number, the amount you make on an ordinary job.

Gord: On an ordinary job…

Anny: And for the same time, compare the two. What is left?

Gord: It would be, not double, but maybe a third more than another job.

Anny: Even with all the money you lost?

Gord: Yah. Very well paying job.

Anny: No but it is simply, it is not that. We also have a way of keeping our income at a certain level. And that is what I want to check, but no.

Gord: No, like even the last three days that I worked. They were all double time days. Instead of making $40 per hour, I was making $80 per hour, 12-hour days. So that is big money. So that is like $600 a day in my pocket after taxes and expenses and everything. So that was really good money and it could have carried on like that.

And he said, the foreman said well my supervisor does not really want to give you a layoff because he just put in another request for 16 people. And so I said whether he gives it to me or not, I will have to go. So I had to sign a special form and that, but you know, that was a real kick in the butt for me to leave there. I had to do what I had to do. Just because I chose the wrong words Oh my Lord..

Anny: Are we not clever?

Gord: No.

Anny: I think we are priceless. I really do.

Gord: And I am still very tight in here. And it is different than other times. Like other times it is right in the lungs, but it is right in here. And sometimes just a simple cough would make me feel better temporary.

<u>The perfect timing to go for the mental block, the cause of it all.</u>

Anny: Just put hands there. There is a place over there now, huh.

Now I know you do not like it, but with each inhale, you will find that feeling there getting stronger and stronger. I know you do not like it. That is right, so go into that feeling. I know you do not like it. But just for now, let that feeling over there become stronger and stronger with each inhale. And with each exhale, let that feeling go way back in time, way way way back in time, way back to whatever it feels, not you, it feels started the whole thing. The feeling, not you. The first thing that comes to you, even if it does not make sense at all to you. Go inside there. Go inside. That feeling knows when it started. It knows very well when it started. Go in there.

Gord: Oh, it started with the oily smell.

Anny: No that is your head talking. But the oily smell, okay, let us go for the oily smell. The oily smell, the oily smell. Take some slow deep breath and as you exhale, go into the oily smells and with each exhale, you are sliding back in time, sliding back in time to that oily smell, oily smell, sliding back to whatever it is way back in time, way back in time, that oily smell, first thing that came to you.

Gord: I am just thinking horses for some reason, I do not know.

Anny: That is okay. And how old are you with that feeling?

Gord: That was just this year.

Anny: You see you are in your head.

Gord: I am in my head I do not know.

Anny: Yes, you tried to think where it is, instead of letting that feeling tell you where it is. The feeling knows, the feeling knows.

Gord: I do not know how to get there.

Anny: Well that is because you cannot think and a feeling does not talk. Um hum, so become aware of your lungs now, your lungs.

Gord: It is right up here.

Anny: They are expanding and contracting, expanding and contracting in a beautiful rhythmic manner and each breathe that you take makes you go deeper and deeper, deeper and deeper into relaxation and as your breath flows, as it comes, as it goes, notice that the sensation is a little cooler when you breathe in than when you breathe out, just a little cooler. Just a little cooler.

That is right. As I am asking for your protection and your well being I say God, please allow only good things to come to Gord.
And for this blessing we give thanks.

And now you ask to be placed into the protection of your very own light, your spark of life. It is like a mini sun in your chest. Some people can see it. Some people can feel it. Some people simply know it is there. That light of yours, that very beautiful light of yours, let it shine, let it shine, let it shine throughout every cell of your body, throughout your aura, cleansing your body, cleansing your aura, strengthening your body, strengthening your aura. Extending itself at one arm's length above you, beneath you, at each side of you, in front of you and behind you and mentally repeat with me, this is my body, this is my space. Only light can come to me. Only light can come from me. Only my light can be here.

And as you take a slow deep breath and exhale, find yourself in a place that suggests relaxation to you. That is right.

A place that suggests relaxation to you. Something that you really enjoy. And in that place, you will discover a very beautiful staircase. Wherever you are, you will discover some things. A staircase you did not know was there. It is a staircase, absolutely beautiful and as you are discovering that staircase, you decide to go down the stairs. It is so beautiful.

So as you take a slow deep breath and exhale, you start to go down the stairs, one step at a time, one step at a time and you notice there are only ten steps and it is absolutely gorgeous. So here you are going down the stairs one step at a time, knowing that with each step down, you are going deeper and deeper and deeper into relaxation. Deeper and deeper and deeper into relaxation.

That is right. And as you go deeper and deeper into relaxation, going down the stairs one step at a time, that is right, one step at a time, you are finding also that you are getting younger and smaller, smaller and younger. Younger and smaller, smaller and younger with each step down. Each step down.

And when you are at the bottom of the stairs, you find yourself very small, very very small, very small. And you feel very comfortable. Very very small and very comfortable. It is as if though you were in your Mother's womb. It is as if though you were in your Mother's womb. Relaxed, relaxed, relaxed, that is right. So relaxed, so relaxed. That is right, feeling great in every way. So enjoy the place, enjoy feeling very very small in your Mother's womb. Just be there, be there, be there.

And as you take a slow deep breath and exhale, you will find that as something is happening wherever you are and there is a feeling there in your chest, there is a feeling in your chest and you are going to become aware of what is creating such a feeling in your chest. Trust what comes to your awareness, that feeling on your chest there. First thing that comes to you, even if it does not make sense to you.

Gord: Aw, my Mom is smoking.

Anny: Is that right. Your Mother is smoking. Your Mother is smoking. And how does it feel that your Mother is smoking?

Gord: Well, it is uncomfortable.

Anny: And where are you as your Mother is smoking? Trust what comes even if it does not make sense to you.

Gord: By the kitchen, she is doing some sewing.

Anny: By the kitchen. And as you are taking a slow deep breath and exhale, you are going to rewind the movie of time to before that happens. How do you feel?

Gord: I feel okay.

Anny: Okay. And then as you take a slow deep breath and exhale, you are going to become very much aware of what makes you comfortable before she smokes. What does she do? Trust what comes, always, even if it does not make sense.

Gord: I do not understand what you want.

Anny: I want to know what is she doing? What are you doing before she is by the kitchen smoking?

Gord: Smoking somewhere else. Always smoking.

Anny: Always smoking. And when she is smoking, what is it that she does not do?

Gord: She does not care.

Anny: How do you feel when she smokes?

Gord: Ah, I feel it is dirty. I do not know how I feel.

Anny: She knew she should not be smocking.

Gord: What a waste of money. But then at that age...

Anny: I was going to say, but I am talking about Gord then. What did Gord then felt he was missing when his Mother was smoking?

Gord: Her attention.

Anny: So what would you do to have her attention when she was smoking?

Gord: I would get just real close and tug at her I guess.

Anny: And would that work?

Gord: Oh yah, she would always give me a hug.

Anny: So as you take a slow deep breath and exhale, you are going to advance for the first time that you feel that thing in your chest.

Gord: Aw, that was in my teens, early teens.

Anny: What was happening?

Gord: Oh again, that was that story from before when I was up the river and started getting sick.

Anny: But then what did you wish you would do?

Gord: But what would I wish I would do – get rid of that feeling.

Anny: Yah, no no, I am not talking about that. Just like when your Mother was smoking, you felt like you were missing her attention.

Gord: I just wish I was with her.

Anny: Hum?

Gord: At that time I wish I was with her, just that was the only thing on my mind was when I was feeling terrible like that.

Anny: When feeling terrible, feeling terrible, wanting your Mother huh? And then what would you do? You were feeling terrible like that, you wanted your Mother and then?

Gord: At that time we turned the boat around and we headed back.

Anny: But as you take a slow deep breath and exhale, go back to when you were a little boy there and the Mother was smoking.

Gord: Okay.

Anny: I am going to ask you to look at something in your mind there and the feelings also. What do you do each time you want your Mom's attention?

Gord: I would go climb up on her.

Anny: Take a deep breath and as you exhale, you are going to advance to when you started to use health as an excuse. First thing that came.

Gord: I am at a doctor's office getting needles.

Anny: And who would drive you there or take you there?

Gord: Well, my brother and I we would walk there after school.

Anny: And then what would happen after that?

Gord: And then we would just play, do our normal thing.

Anny: Your brother huh. Which brother is that, older or younger?

Gord: The younger one.

Anny: The younger one huh. So together you would go there. And how did you feel both together doing that?

Gord: Companion I guess, someone to play with. Just company going there, instead of going to a doctor's office by myself.

Anny: What would happen if you went to the doctor's office yourself? Go back then.

Gord: It would be okay. It would be okay. No problem with it.

Anny: But how would you feel that you have to go alone?

Gord: It would not bother me.

Anny: Oh yah? As you take a slow deep breath and exhale, go back and forth in your life, back and forth, back and forth and you will become very much aware of when you feel you want companionship or whatever. There is a feeling there. Um hum. When you feel terrible, you wanted your Mother, so what did you do to get your Mother?

Gord: I would go get her attention.

Anny: So what do you do – I am going to ask you. You know what, that reminds me of a very good friend of mine who is a therapist. She is using something very different. She is very good and what happened is here she gets a call from someone who has asthma and allergy attacks,

And she removes it. No hypnosis. Totally different, but you do not go for what for, what is so nice about it. Not at all, you just remove it. So two months later the lady called, she said to my friend, is there any way she can have it back. Well said my friend, what is it?. She is missing all the attention she is getting and so guess what, it is about two months later and she asked my friend to get it back. And do you know what my friend told her? Keep thinking about it and you will get it back.

Gord: Yah, just like you are telling me.

Anny: Yes.

Gord: But I try not to think about it.

Anny: The thing is not thinking about it is the problem.

Gord: Not thinking about it?

Anny: It is one of the reasons you are using it for. And you keep saying you wanted your Mother and here she is still smoking. Oh, so what do you do to get her attention. You started that very young and it is the attention of a very young woman. So what are you after with Suzy, is your wife name, right? What are you after with her?

Gord: A companion.

Anny: And how do you feel when you are away then?

Gord: Well a little bit lonesome.

Anny: Lonesome. And how lonesome were you feeling when you went to Fort McMurray?

Gord: I was not really away that long to get that lonesome.

Anny: How did you feel that you had your birthday over there?

Gord: I was not too thrilled with it, but we did have birthday cake the day before we left and that sort of stuff. I have had worst birthdays.

Anny: And how did you feel then?

Gord: Not good Not good..

Anny: You see, I am doing everything for you to access the feeling, but you are making sure you are not going there. You think....

Gord: It is not on purpose.

Anny: I know that. And I am wondering how old you were when you discovered it works. Because I found out something that aw, what is that. But after that the second time, hey, I can use it for that. The first time is always, what is that, the second time, hum.

Gord: You know the time that I really. One I can really think of is when I am home at Kingston and quite often my dog likes cheese and I had put it in my teeth and he would come and take it away. And one day it just stuffed me up.

Anny: Who said anything about you doing that with your dog?

Gord: What feeding him that way? It is just a trick sort of a thing.

Anny: The thing is anybody saw you doing that?

Gord: No, after...

Anny: What was said?

Gord: Maybe the first time I did it alone or if there was somebody there. I do not know but I may have brought it up watch what my dog will do. He will take this from me. It was sort of – I cannot remember specifically but it would have been a funny thing to see and then all of a sudden one day it stuffed me up. Another earlier time getting stuffed up was farmer neighbors of mine, we had a sleepover in the barn. Well about 2:00 in the morning I am so badly stuffed up from the hay and everything, I had to go home. Another time I was stuffed up, another time on the farm again, the horses, the horses were just awful. As much as I like them, such a majestic animal, and then would just stuff me up.

Anny: What happened then?

Gord: Well, I would feel like I had a flu for the next day.

Anny: What do you do?

Gord: Go home eventually.

Anny: Go home every time. You were in Fort McMurray, huh, go home.

Gord: Yah.

Anny: So take a deep breathe now and as you exhale, close your eyes and go back to the hay thing, the farm there and the sleepover, what time of the day was it – you had to go home?

Gord: Two or three.

Anny: About two in the morning and you had to go home and compare that experience to Fort McMurray?

Gord: Very much parallel to each other.

Anny: And how old were you when you were on the hay there?

Gord: Fifteen, sixteen or seventeen.

Anny: Can you put the fifteen-year-old in front of you here?

Gord: More like seventeen, I guess.

Anny: Well the seventeen year old, put him in front of you and ask him to let you know from the bottom of his heart that makes him, how did he feel about the whole situation that made him decide to go home?

Gord: I was really having fun. I did not want to go home but because I could not breathe, I knew I had to go somewhere different.

Anny: So take a deep breathe and ask the seventeen year old, the teenager, what was the not being able to breathe all about? What is it that he could not take? What is it that you cannot take?

Gord: Just all the dust in the air. All the dust in the air. It is not that I missed Mom, and had to go back or anything like that.

Anny: Well where did you go?

Gord: Well I did go home.

Anny: Um hum and what happened there, two o'clock in the morning?

Gord: Oh there I was away from all the hay.

Anny: I am talking about what happened at home when you got home?

Gord: I cannot recall.

Anny: Did you make sure that everybody was surprised to see you there in the morning and wake up the whole place or whatever?

Gord: They would definitely be surprised to see me at home. They would figure I would be gone all night. I cannot remember if I woke up anybody up when I got home. Because at that time, there were no inhalers that I know of.

Anny: Now become aware of your lungs again. Your lungs, they are expanding and contracting, expanding and contracting in a beautiful rhythmic manner. And every breath that you take makes you go deeper and deeper and deeper into relaxation. And as you breath flows, as it comes, as it goes, notice that the sensation is a little cooler when you breathe in than when you breathe out. Just a little cooler. Just a little cooler. And with each exhale, you find yourself getting younger and smaller, smaller and younger, feeling great, feeling great to be Gord. Way back, way back, feeling great to be Gord.

As you go deeper and deeper and deeper into relaxation. Feeling so great, truly enjoying being Gord. Really enjoying it. Truly, it feels so great to be Gord. That is right and when you are there, feeling great, and when you are there whatever is going on, simply nod.

Thank you. Just enjoy that feeling. Just enjoy that feeling of feeling so great. Feeling so great and breathe it in. It feels so great, just breathe in that feeling. Breathe in that feeling. It feels so great. It feels so great. So relaxed, so comfortable. And as you take a slow deep breath and exhale, be there, be there. And become very much aware and who has all the attention at home. Who has all the attention at home? First thing that came. Whose getting all the attention at home?

Gord: Well, I was thinking me. It was sort of shared between my brother and me.

Anny: So how did it feel that you were sharing between your brother and you? How did that feel that you had to share?

Gord: It did not bother me, because I had two parents and if I did not get attention from one, I had be the other I guess.

Anny: So what did you do to get attention? Be very much aware of that.

Gord: Go sit on their lap.

Anny: And as you take a slow deep breath and exhale, you are going to get to a point where you are going to sit on their lap and it is outdated so to speak. So what do you do then?

Gord: What do I do for attention?

Anny: Yup. Well, have a look at what your brother does for attention.

Gord: Well, he was the more quiet one but he used to like to bug me.

Anny: What is he doing to get attention. Have a look.

Gord: At that age, he was more intellectual.

Anny: And what was he doing for attention?

Gord: I just see him sitting there watching T.V. being a good boy.

Anny: So what was his idea then to also needing shots and going with you?

Gord: No, he did not. That was my younger brother that needed the shots. The older one did not.

Anny: But the thing is how come you focus on your older brother when I ask who has attention at home?

Gord: Because the younger one was not there yet.

Anny: Oh, and how old were you when the younger one came?

Gord: I was about six.

Anny: And how did it feel?

Gord: To have a younger brother come? I was excited.

Anny: And whose getting all the attention?

Gord: Well the baby gets more attention.

Anny: So what did you do to get attention?

Gord: Well there was no lack of attention.

Anny: No, you made sure there was not huh. If you were a stranger watching Gord and his older brother and a baby in the house, how did it feel to not being the baby any more?

Gord: A little bit more time to myself.

Anny: No more being the baby.

Gord: I have to do more stuff for myself.

Anny: So take a deep breathe now and together with six year old Gord who is no longer the baby, I would like you to go back and forth, back and forth and become very much aware of how you behave now at what age are you functioning now. Not being comfortable any more in your chest when you are about to lay down. Not comfortable when there is smile. That is right, how old are you? Pretend you are a total stranger observing all this.

Gord: The only thing I see is on that farm but it was years before that I had allergies. I cannot recall.

Anny: The feeling knows.

Gord: Pardon me?

Anny: The feeling has it all. You know your subconscious mind knows exactly what you are doing. It knows exactly and I am asking your subconscious mind to do it's perfect job and do it now so that at the most unexpected time, you discover what is so nice about it. The whole situation. What is so nice about it and how you are not letting it go and then open your eyes.

Anny: Gord, if you had a friend that goes through the same thing as you, what would you tell him?

Gord: Go see Anny.

Anny: Thank you.

Okay, Gord I learned a long time ago, when you do it more than twice there is because there is a perceived benefit from it. So what are you using it for?

Gord: I really do not know Anny. You make me feel like it is attention or something. But I cannot see that.

Anny: It came up before. It is not Gord now that wants attention.

Gord: Yah, I had lots of attention. I was always doing stuff.

Anny: Yah, but then you always managed to go home, huh?

Gord: Well, yah, home is where you have to go home at the end of the day. Home is your kind of sanctuary sort of thing.

Anny: Hum, you are saying that sort of thing in a certain way there. How do you feel that you have to go where you have to go after today?

Gord: It is a good place for me to go.

Anny: Okay, what do you do to be welcomed?

Gord: I greet everybody when I come home. Hugs and all that sort of stuff. It is just a good place to be. I have no problem going home.

Anny: When you were a little boy, go back to when you decide going home is a good place to be, which is a good thing by the way. Going home is a good place to be. By the way, I do not remember that because I do not have the paper. Are your parents still living?

Gord: My Mother is. My Father died about ten years ago.

Anny: Close your eyes and what would happen if you would go there and have the same scenario as if you were a little boy, what would happen then?

Gord: If I go where?

Anny: In your Mother's place, the same scenario as before, as a teenager, how would she respond?

Gord: You mean when I would be stuffed up as a teenager?

Anny: Yes.

Gord: Well, she would try and find a solution for it. You know, try to play doctor a little bit, try to give me either a hot drink or something.

Anny: And what would happen then?

Gord: I would get to feeling better. Being home, away from the problem.

Anny: Being away from the problem, what problem are you talking about?

Gord: Well at the farm, in the dust and that around the horses, cows, everything. I would come home where I could breathe.

Anny: So when you left Fort McMurray, compare that to the feelings you had with that feeling there. So how old are you in that performance?

Gord: With the horses and that?

Anny: With everything now. When you came back from Fort McMurray there, how old were you really in that whole situation?

Gord: Fifty-three.

Anny: Yah, going what? Seventeen. Fifteen, six years old. There is a younger Gord there that you better get ahold of.

Gord: For what?

Anny: Hey by the way, how old is your oldest son?

Gord: Eighteen.

Anny: Since when?

Gord: Since last month.

Anny: Okay so he was seventeen. And that horse thing it was seventeen, eighteen. Because children trigger parents major. So what was going on at that time in your life that you were doing all that stuff.

Going back home away from the problem. I am not talking about the dust and everything, I am talking about what was the problem. Close your eyes. What was causing your problems in your life then? What was causing problems in your life then?

Gord: There is a lot of stress at school.

Anny: Lots of stress at school.

Gord: Again, I would always be sick. Always from dust and whatever, I would always be sneezing and blowing my nose and running nose and that got to me and I was just sickly.

Anny: And what was nice about being sickly?

Gord: Nothing.

Anny: Ah ah ah, I am talking to the teenager.

Gord: There was nothing. I cannot see anything, no benefit to it.

Anny: No girlfriend, no nothing?

Gord: Ah, there were at times.

Anny: And exams and things like that?

Gord: Ah exams.

Anny: Well you have to pass exams, write exams and everything.

Gord: Yah, well I was not too interested in that.

Anny: What were you interested in?

Gord: Just having fun.

Anny: Just having fun. And as you take a slow deep breath and exhale, have a look at your son. What is going on in his life and compare it to yours.

Gord: He seems to be a little bit more together than I was. I think he is not really into the partying. He has a steady girlfriend you know. If I look at him and I look at myself, I would say he is doing quite well.

Anny: Okay. So what were you avoiding?

Gord: When, when I was a teenager?

Anny: As a teenager.

Gord: I do not know if I was avoiding anything.

Anny: What?

Gord: I do not know if I was avoiding anything.

Anny: What is it that you could not do because of all that physical condition?

Gord: Just could not do anything that took any physical really for instance, I could think of one time that really affected me. I had to shovel a bunch of sand into wheelbarrows and move it somewhere else. And that is when I took notice. My older brother, who I thought I could outdo him no problem. But I was so quick to lose energy, where he just went on and on.

Anny: Okay, so sickly huh. So take a deep breath now Gord and as you exhale listen to the humming of the ventilation system and as you are listening to the humming of the ventilation system you can feel yourself becoming very very relaxed and your hands are getting so heavy, so heavy there on your chest that they are sliding down, sliding down into your lap. That is right, sliding down, sliding down, sliding down, into your lap.

That is right. Becoming so relaxed and your hands are getting so heavy and the deeper the relaxation the heavier your hands and the heavier your hands, the faster they are sliding down on your lap. That is right, that is right. Going deeper and deeper into relaxation and this time you find yourself in a very fancy place.

<u>"Winging" The Building Induction</u>

Very very fancy place. With a very unique elevator. Fancy and unique elevator. Very fancy place and quite a unique elevator and as you take a slow deep breath and exhale, you step on the elevator. You are really high and the elevator is going to go down, down. So you call up the elevator, step into it and then push floor number one. The first floor and you are relaxing and since this elevator is going slowly down, down down and you notice that each floor number is the same than your age and as you go down, the ages are going smaller and smaller of course.
So you get to 50, 49, 48.

The elevator is going down, down and will stop at whatever it was that made you decide to be sickly. You are going to find that elevator is going to stop at that age. That is right. The time you decided to be sickly.

That is right. And it will not make sense to you. As you go deeper and deeper into relaxation. And when the elevator stops, simply nod. All right. What age did it stop at?

Gord: Does not make sense, but twenty-seven.

Anny: That is okay. But twenty-seven, twenty-seven. Step out of the elevator and you will find at whatever it is that you got you to decide to be sickly. Whatever it is it is there on that floor, floor twenty-seven. And it will not make sense to you.

Gord: That is when I moved out west.

Anny: That is when you moved out west.

Gord: But I was sickly before that.

Anny: I am not talking about that, just stay there. Moved out west. Is that right, and what is happening there. Moving out west. How did that feel to move?

Gord: It felt good, good. All the work was out here at the time.

Anny: Yah which is true, but, there is two sides to every coin. What was the other side?

Gord: Well, I missed my family.

Anny: Um hum. So stay there yah. So what is that twenty-seven year old Gord decided to be sick. Trust it, it will not make sense to you and it is fine. By being sickly, what does that remind him of?

Gord: Oh, it is funny. Around that same time when I was twenty-seven, all these symptoms sort of disappeared. Until I was maybe five or six years I do not remember any real problems.

Anny: Five, six years huh. So about thirty-three. So take a deep breathe and as you exhale, advance to thirty-three and what happened that got it back on? First thing that came to you.

Gord: Well, I had my little dog again.

Anny: What happened at thirty-three?

Gord: I still had allergies towards him.

Anny: Yah but that still does not tell me what is going on in your life at thirty-three.

Gord: What is going on in my life at thirty-three? Well just a lot of partying was going on.

Anny: How old were you when you got married?

Gord: Thirty-four, thirty-five.

Anny: When did you meet Suzy?

Gord: In 87.

Anny: In 87?

Gord: Yes.

Anny: And you are 54. You were 33. What is that women trigger that in you?

Gord: Pardon me.

Anny: What is that women trigger that sickly kid in you?

Take a deep breath and as you exhale go back to that very young, six, seven, eight, whatever and ask the very young Gord that when you started to meet Suzy, you started to be sick again? Ask the young lad, he will tell you. The younger one yah. And it will not make sense to you.

Gord: No, he is not answering.

Anny: Give him a hug and say now come on.

Gord: I cannot get anything.

Anny: Ask him to let you know what is it that he does not want to tell you? Ask the young boy there, what is that he does not want to tell you?

Gord: I cannot get it. I cannot get anything out of him.

Anny: Can he draw you something. If he does not want to tell you, can he draw it, or make a movie, give you a movie?

Gord: He is just there. He is just like a picture, he is not moving or anything.

Anny: Is it not the time he got a little baby brother? Give him a hug. So what decision did he make about his Mother? What decision did he make about his Mother?

Gord: She was always busy.

Anny: And how did you feel about that?

Gord: I felt that was something that just had to be done. As much as I would like...

Anny: So who was doing everything?

Gord: Mother.

Anny: And what are you doing to make sure it was her? I am talking to the young one huh.

Gord: Always being there.

Anny: How does that feel?

Gord: It feels okay. I know I am never too far from her. Even though she was occupied at times, I will still have my time.

Anny: So as you take a slow deep breath and exhale, compare that to what is going on at home now.

Gord: I guess much the same thing.

Anny: Is not that interesting. So now how old are you now in your behaviour, in your feelings?

Gord: Six years old. Yah.

Anny: So that is why you are feeling what is around you?

Gord: Just do not tell Suzy.

Anny: No I do not say anything to anybody. So now as you take a slow deep breathe now, together with the young six years old, back in your life, back and forth, back and forth and have a good sense of humour about it, a very good sense of humour about it. It makes such a difference to have a good laugh about it.

Gord: Yah, there is a lot of parallels there.

Anny: Uh huh. So have a good sense of humour about that. So ask the younger lad what was the nicest thing about it at six years old? What is the nicest thing about it?

Gord: All play.

Anny: Give him a hug. And I am going to ask him to have a good look at you. Here you are a good 45 years later. Ask him to look at you and explain to him something and at this point in your life. You can play if you want to and you can work if you want to. And you can feel good all the time if you want. Make sure you tell him that you understand how come he used all that sickness. You understand that.

Gord: Say that again.

Anny: Tell him that you understand how come you had to be sick all the time. No shoveling, no nothing, is it not that great!

Give him a hug and tell him that is very smart of him. It is, you say what you want. The thing is now you know your interests are different. You like to play but also like to do other things too. Explain to him that welding is like playing because you like it so much. So explain to him that welding is like playing. It can make things, cut things, you can put things together, you can dismantle. You can do all kinds of things. It is great. It is almost like a Lego thing there. You know you can put it together, take it apart. Explain that to the guy, the young lad. It is okay to play, it is okay to weld. Just explain to him the joy of what you are doing. And how does that feel Gord? How does it feel?

Gord: Oh it feels, I will let him know about it.

Anny: So breath in that pleasure of doing. Hey and explain to him to top it off you are paid for it. Can you imagine? Paid to do what you like to do. Just breathe it in, breathe it in. So it is all right to be fine all the time.

And something is coming to mind.

He likes to play? So how does it feel to play sick because that is about the size of it.

Ask him if he ever wanted to be an actor. It is a game, is it not? He is pretty good at it, huh. But you are better and well and when you feel that the young lad has understood, simply nod.

The hand closure and integration of the two parts method

Okay, so now then in one hand let the part of you who knows how to breathe easily at all times, let that part come into one of your hands and when it is there, simply turn it up, so that I know that you are holding it. Okay.

Gord: Let the part of me that know…..

Anny: How to breathe easily at all times.

At this point, the recording was full and stopped. The session continued on and the result: The asthma is completely gone now.

Questions About Bill's Session

- Question 1 -

- Question 2 -

- Question 3 -

- Question 4 -

- Question 5 -

Transcript: Fire Accident, The Sacred Vow

August 14, 2008
Filmed Private Session Demonstration

It was the last day of HYP 204.
As the class was leaving for lunch, I noticed a question mark over every student's head, wondering how to apply all the "tools" they had in their toolbox.

I then decided to do a demonstration.

When they came back from lunch, I explained I was going to do a session demonstration, having no idea what "tools" I was going to use, simply following the needs of a client.

Students share very little personal information with me. Therefore, knowing only that he was in a fire accident, I asked Bill if he would agree to be a volunteer. Yes, was his answer.

Anny: Alright, now. Okay Bill, that – those burns, how long ago?

Bill: Well, 1985, 1986. I think '85.

Anny: 1985?

Bill: '85. About 23 years ago.

Anny: Okay, thank you, about 23 years ago.

Bill: Mm-hmm.

Anny: Okay, hmm. How much do you remember of it all?

Bill: Some of it is very, very clear.

Anny: Tell me which one is clear?

Bill: Um, you know I am not even sure I can actually recall the ignition moment. I know what I was doing. Um, I was refilling a wood alcohol burner, it was underneath the fondue, and I was filling it from-

Anny: What type of fondue?

Bill: Um, well just a pot,

Anny: What did you put in there?
Bill: Oh, we had vegetables, and we had little cubes of meat that we were cooking on skewers in the fondue.

Anny: Okay, so it was, in there it was oil in there or water?

Bill: Oil.

Anny: Oil, okay, so it was, now I understand what you mean, because you can do a lot of things with it, so I did not know what it was. Okay, so you were cooking –

Bill: In the hot oil.

Anny: In the hot oil.

Bill: And in order to keep that going, because it was on the kitchen table, there is a little wood alcohol burner that goes underneath it, just to keep it hot.

Anny: Yes.

Bill: And, it went out. At least I thought it went out, I am pretty sure it went out. But anyway, so, there is no flame left there. And so, my friend - we were at my friend's place, and he had a jug, a gallon jug of wood alcohol. So I took the little burner out and I poured the fuel into the burner. And that is when, I kind of turned into a candle. Because, as I was pouring it, it did not explode, it just moved up,

Anny: Yes.

Bill: And so, it just moved up, the fuel moved up my hand, then the whole jug was on fire,

Anny: Mm-hmm!

Bill: Some must have splashed on my clothes, because then my shirt was on fire, and everything was just turning into,

Anny: Mm-hmm.

Bill: Everything was on fire. And um, I was behind the table at the time, and I had my three small children there, my wife,

Anny: How old were they?

Bill: Uh, John was 4, Joy was 3, and Alicia was just a baby, she was just one.

Anny: Okay.

Bill: So, I am behind the table and all of a sudden everything is on fire, and in fact the curtains are starting to catch on fire, and the table is on fire, everything is on fire. So I had to get out of there, right now, and I could not just throw the thing, so I walked around the back of the side of the table, carrying this jug of flaming wood alcohol, and I made it out the back door of the kitchen.

Anny: Okay.

Bill: Uh, that part is fairly, fairly clear. Uh, after that, um, shock sets in really, really quick, and some of the next part gets kind of, uh not too clear.

Anny: Okay.

Bill: Uh, some very very clear moments are, I remember looking down at my hands, and saying, "Oh, gee I really should take off these gloves." Except the deal was, I was not wearing gloves. It was my skin, it looked like grey gloves. At any rate, my little boy was really, really sharp. He scooted under the table, he ran to the neighbors, he said, "The house is on fire, my daddy is on fire, we need help!" Four years old, and so,

Anny: Is that your oldest son?

Bill: Ya, my only son.

Anny: Uh-huh. Is that the son that you would do anything for him?

Bill: You betcha. You betcha.

Anny: Uh-huh.

Bill: I would do anything for all of them.

Anny: Ya, but that one,

Bill: I have done the most for him.

Anny: Uh-huh.

Bill: It is true.

Anny: You smile.

Bill: Ya!

Anny: Okay. Mm-hmm.

Bill: So anyway, I got bundled off to the hospital. This was in Peace River, which at that time was population maybe 6000. And I remember a doctor kind of walking around me, as if he was afraid to touch me. It was just beyond what he,

Anny: Ever saw.

Bill: Ever saw, or could handle. Because you know, my skin was charred, my shirt was embedded,

Anny: Oh ya!

Bill: It melted, I was wearing 65/35 polyester. Just great fuel.

Anny: Uh-huh.

Bill: So this is all embedded in my chest area, it was all burned and charred. My head is already starting to swell, and it is getting bigger. My ears are drooping off and they look like a pig roast.

Anny: Okay.

Bill: And uh, so he just did not know what to do with me, and he, so they bundled me off to STARS and sent me to the U of A Hospital, where I spent 6 weeks in the burn unit. And the next 2 years in recovery, really. I actually went back to work within 4 months, believe it or not. I was pretty determined I was going back to work. But having to wear the uh, the tight burn dressings, that keep your scars from raising,

Anny: Mm-hmm!

Bill: It is like you are in, if you can imagine, the heaviest support hose you have ever had.

Anny: Mm-hmm.

Bill: Times 20, to just keep you sucked in, keep the scars flat. And you know, other than that, itch was kind of a big deal, because if you ever burn yourself, you know how much it itches, as it heals, and if you can imagine 50% of the body being itchy all at once, it was a little bit of itch there. Um, and probably within, ah I mean, there were skin grafts, I do remember some of the hospitalization. I remember some of, well hallucinations.

Anny: Tell me about that.

Bill: Well, they give you a lot of drugs to keep down the pain. And you are already in pain, which is distorting reality for you. Plus, they give you drugs, and you are in shock anyway, so I remember one day lying in the hospital bed, and uh, floating up at the ceiling,

Anny: Of course.

Bill: Almost touching the ceiling.

Anny: And how did you feel then?

Bill: Oh I did not like that at all. It was really hot up there, and nasty. And I just wanted, let me out of here, let me down.

Anny: Is I not that interesting?

Bill: I did not like that at all. Other hallucinations, I would be talking to someone and it would be, well I was lecturing the Legislature on the dangers of fondues and I was warning them that in this very hospital, there were 200 of them sitting in their basement, just waiting to make trouble for somebody.

Anny: Okay, hey -

Bill: Um, hallucinations – my mom brought me some borscht, some soup. I said, "you know how many Ukrainians have died from eating that stuff?" She is just bringing me soup…

Anny: (Laughing)

Bill: And a friend, a very, very good friend I was really angry with because he had not come to see me even once. And that was after weeks of being in there, and then I was told he had actually been there every day. So, a lot of distortions.

Anny: Ya, lots of distortions.

Bill: Ya.

Anny: Okay, now,

Bill: And lots of pain, with the grafting. You know, I mean they just slice it off your leg and then staple it onto where you need it.

Anny: They did a good job!

Bill: They did, they did, a really decent job.

Anny: They really did a very good job.

Bill: It keeps me together, um,

Anny: Repeat that again!

Bill: It is serving me well, it keeps me together. If you do not have skin on top of you-

Anny: It keeps you together!

Bill: Well it covers me up. It keeps infection from-

Anny: You know what I am saying. It keeps you together. Okay, which – you understand me,

Bill: I am not sure I understand what you are saying.

Anny: Well, you will see.
Bill: Okay.

Anny: Now, that is 23 years ago.
Mm-hmm. What did you do to have peace of mind about that?

Bill: At first, one of the questions I asked of the doctor, I said, "*Well, when will I be normal again?*"

Anny: And what did they say?

Bill: The fact of it is, he could not really answer that, he kind of sloughed it away. He said, "*Well, I is really not gonna be like it used to be, it is not ever, like normal, again.*"

Anny: Oh.

Bill: How did I come to peace with the whole thing? I think at first, I was really quite self-conscious about my appearance. And as are a lot of people who have burns, or fresh deformity of some sort, quite self-conscious. And then, I joined the group called the Alberta Burn Rehabilitation Society. They are a lot of people there, these are old burns, fresh burns, whatever. And uh, it was a place where, we sort of all had that one, common experience.

Anny: Mm-hmm.

Bill: And ah, this was not a moan and groan group. This was a group whose motto is "I am not a victim, I am a survivor." And, so they were really a strong help, during that first period. So, I did some socialization with them. Um, how did I first come to peace with it?

You know, at first I would wear long shorts and shirts, if at all, sort of hid them away, if you will. And after a while the whole idea just got stale, of having to be all mussed and fussed up about. And I think the largest part is I just kind of let it go, and I do not notice it so much anymore, and I really believe the first thing that anyone sees of you, after your body shape, is your smile. And I know that there are people,

Anny: Well, you know that is true. I never thought about it, but -

Bill: It is,

Anny: That is true!

Bill: And there are people who I um, have known me for a long time, and we have not discussed it, and they have not even noticed it. So, it is fairly obvious, but lots of people have – and the deal is, it is not a big deal for them, it does not, in any way make our relationship any different.

Anny: You know, I find it very interesting what you say, because you say is very obvious. You know what, I did not even know. And I never thought what it is, that is all, except when you start to look at the nails. I said, okay, what is happening with the nails? So, what emotion is keeping it there?

Bill: Well, I do not know about emotion, but as soon as you suggested this session this morning, I thought back to what I just told you, *when will this all be normal again?* And I thought of that doctor's words and him saying *well, I hate to break it to you but it is never going to be normal.*

Anny: According to who?

Bill: What do you mean by that?

Anny: Where does it come, the idea that it will never be normal again? Where does he get that idea? Where did he get it?

Bill: Well, his science, well from the doctor. And his science is, because you study it up a bit, you know, you have ah, I studied it up, and what they have done is taken a thin layer of skin,
Anny: Mm-hmm.

Bill: Right, they have put it on, say they put it onto my hands, so it is just a thin layer, not the full depth, or else I would not have anything back there. So, it is different from other people's skin, because it is only that thin layer. For example, there will be no, there are no hair follicles here, there are no sweat glands here, um
Oh no,

Anny: You are teaching something, according to you, the doctor. And nothing else.

Bill: If nothing else, I guess maybe I just assumed, okay, the skin is not the same anymore, I just assume all this is damage from that burn, and that part of it just is.

Anny: Mm-hmm. So, according to you, Bill, what would fix it? What would allow it to be okay according to you? What is required so that those nails are the way they were intended to be?

Bill: Well the first thing that would have to happen is I would have to cancel that message from that doctor, which says that they cannot be.

Anny: Yes, it can be, if you want. Whose life is it, yours or the doctors?

Bill: Mine.

Anny: That is it. Who is body is it? What is the intelligence within you that kept you the way you are? Talk about a leading question! (laughing) Where is the intelligence that made you, that keeps you alive and so forth? Where is it?

Bill: Well, I think that I accepted what that doctor had to say as the way it is going to be, and I never even suspected that I could do anything about it.

Anny: Okay, which I do understand.

Bill: I should say, I never suspected until lately that I could do something about it.

Anny: Oh, yes. Now, there are several things about this, okay, that is why I am smiling. Okay, there are several things about that. Can I see the other nails? Okay.

Bill: I did not manicure them so well for today.

Anny: Ah, you did not know that I would look. Oh, I got you by surprise huh? Okay. Alright.
For you, with your awareness and everything, and as you said, not until lately did you realize that, *well, I did not know, I could do something about that.* Okay, so what I wonder is, according to you, Bill, what is to be done to cancel that?

Bill: Part of that work has actually already been done.

Anny: Excellent.

Bill: Because I understand that doctors are totally, are imperfect, and uh, for a large part, really unaware of the part that our subconscious is playing.

Anny: Okay, Yah.

Bill: And so, you know, instead of accepting what the doctor said, so it must be so, it is more – medical science may be able to help in some way, but I will still be able to make up my own mind on choices. So part of that work has already been done, like I say, cancel that.

Anny: Mm-hmm. So now I would like you to take a slow, deep breath, and as you exhale, close your eyes. And I would like you to be there, I do not know, let us say, a year from now. And you are you know, filing your nails and so forth, because that is a routine we do on a regular base, because they need to be filed and shaped and everything.
And it is normal, your nails are the natural way. The way they were intended to be in the first place. I would like you to be there.

And as you are there, becoming more and more relaxed, more and more at peace, you rewind the movie of time, so to speak, to when the nails were really not nice at all.

And as you take a slow, deep breath, and exhale, advance again to, in a year from now, the nails are the way they are meant to be. And you are going to become very much aware of what did you let go of, by having nails the way they were intended to be? What did you let go of?

And totally trust what comes to your awareness, even if it does not make sense to you at all.

Bill: I think that I just accepted that that is the way it was meant to be.

Anny: Alright, did you accept it?

Bill: That is what happened.

Anny: So being a hypnotherapist, you are going to understand what I mean by saying, "what was the job that you had given those nails, to stay the way they were, for over 20 years? What job did they have? What was their job, to look the way they looked, for a little over 20 years? They have a job, what is it?"

Your subconscious mind is open and very, very receptive to the suggestions you are receiving now. And I am asking your subconscious mind to reveal to you, the job you gave those nails, without really realizing what you did. And the information will come to you, very clearly and at the most unexpected time. Mm-hmm. And the information will be quite surprising to you. That is right. You gave those nails a job. So, take a deep breath, and open your eyes.

Anchoring - Anny's left.

They have a job, what is it? You will get it. You will get it. So now, take a deep breath, and as you exhale, in your mind go into those nails, the nails you want to have, the way they were intended to be. The way they *are* intended to be.

Close your eyes. Go into those nails and talk to them. Explain to them that you learned to be very careful. Also, in your mind, see all those cells, *see them*, and in your mind do or say whatever you feel is appropriate, so that they are vibrating the way they are supposed to. That they are vibrating full of energy, healthy, and with great peace, harmony. In your mind, show them the way you want them to be. The way they were intended to be, with the quality you liked about it, and shape and looks.

Stop Anchoring

Give your apologies to those nails, make sure that they know, the cells know, that you understand them, and explain to them it has been over 20 years now, whatever message they wanted you to get, you got it.

That is right. You got it, and it is okay, you got the message; you learned your lesson, whatever it was that you had to learn. And they can relax, and get back to the way they are intended to be. And then open your eyes.

Bill: (Eyes open)

Anny: So, how do you feel about what we did so far?

Bill: Uh, I feel fine, I had a tingling in my fingers.

Anny: You did?

Bill: Yah, and that feels good, and uh, it kind of put me up to some of the beliefs I had. There is a negative beliefs there – when you asked me, what is that for?

Anny: Yah, what is that for?

Bill: Why do you need them like that? And it seems to me, it is also an acceptance, you know,

Anny: What do you mean by that?

Bill: Well, I is kind of like a, when you put something out, and well, I did not know, other nice, normal fingernails, and well, I have got these kind of gnarly ones, but you know, it is a question to others, do you accept me that way? Right?

Anchoring right.

Anny: Got it. (laughing)

Bill: So maybe that was sort of it, how important is it? Here is my test to other people – how important is it that I match whatever mold that you may have, whatever? So,

Anny: Okay.

Bill: I do not think I need to do that anymore.

Anny: Yah,

Bill: So there is two things going on in my head.

Anny: Oh yes, so take a deep breath now, and as you exhale, go back to you, when you got burned. He is in the hospital. Walk in there. And do whatever is required to have his attention. And ask him, what is going on in his life, that he feels he needs to test the temperature, so to speak, to know if he is accepted or not. What is going on in his life, that he feels that, well, am I ok? Am I going to be accepted for who I am? What is going on in his life, that he requires that confirmation? And I would like to know what was the answer?

Stop anchoring right.

Bill: There are two things going on in my head. One of them was that, even though the kids were small, it was my marriage was already starting to not work very well for either of us; for me or my spouse. And another thing, I was changing careers and going into new, very different kind of work; it was a higher level, and so, that is what was going on.

Anny: Okay. Take a deep breath now, and as you exhale, as him to have a look at you. Does he know, that here you are, 23 years later? And does he know, that by now, you know where you stand with yourself? You know where you stand within yourself. And reassure him, because of how things are now, that it is okay.

Bill: It is really okay.

Anny: What?

Bill: It is really okay.

Anny: Yes, it is really okay.

Bill: It is better now.

Anchoring left

Anny: So, as you take a slow, deep breath, and exhale, ask him to go back a day before that happened with the fondue, and as you are aware of me holding your head,

Emotional Stress Release

I would like you to go from the day before, the day before that happened with the fondue, to review everything that happened, all the way to when you ran out of that house, on fire. And when you are here, let me know.

Bill: (Nods)

Anny: Alright, rewind everything like a VHS in a VCR, all the way to the day before, and when you are back here, let me know.

Bill: (Nods)

Anny: Now I would like you to go a little further back, to whatever, as far as your mind is going to go, and when you are wherever, as far as you have to go, when your mind, as far as your mind wants to go back, let me know.

Bill: Mm-hmm.

Anny: Now, you are going to review everything, all the way back, all the way from - Review everything from there, you are going to review everything to when you got on the helicopter, to go to the U of A Hospital. That is where you went, huh? And when you are in that, you know, flown out by STARS ambulance, let me know. And please say so, so I know you are there. (pause)

Bill: (Nods)

Anny: Rewind everything all the way back to wherever you went. And when you are back there, let me know.

Bill: (Nods)

Anny: Now, as you are going to review it again, from there all the way to when you got flown out by STARS ambulance, I want you this time to become very much aware of what was on your mind, as well as whatever happened. So review everything from there, all the way to when you are flown out by STARS ambulance. And when you are on that, on STARS ambulance, let me know. And you become very much aware of your train of thoughts.

Bill: (Nods)

Anny: Rewind everything again, to as far as you went to. I know it is not very pleasant, but that is the way it goes, back there. And as you take a slow, deep breath, and exhale, you are going to review slowly, everything, all the way to when you asked that doctor, if everything would be back to normal again, and including the doctor's expression, and his answer, and then how you felt about it.

Bill: (Nods)

Anny: Rewind everything to where you were, or maybe even farther back, your mind will know where to go.

Bill: (Nods)

Anny: And now you are going to review it again, and this time you are going to go all the way to now, in this chair.

Bill: (Nods)

Anny: Rewind everything to as far as you went, now listen carefully. You are going to review everything, but this time, stop here; (top of head) at the crucial time in the whole situation. The most traumatic time in the whole situation. And stop here, and tell me when you are there.

Bill: Mm-hmm.

Anny: Okay, now listen carefully, at the speed that I will move my hands from where they are to the top of your head and back where they are now, you are going to stretch the whole thing, from where you stopped, all the way back to the very, as far as you went, and at the same time, from where you stopped, to here in this chair. It is like stretching it. So are you ready? Take a deep breath, and as you exhale, stretch it. That is right. Breathe in, that is right.

Rewind everything again, because we will do it again, all the way to as far as you went. And now review it and stop here, to the most traumatic moment in the whole situation. And keep breathing. Now, we will stretch it again, so take a deep breath, and as you exhale, stretch it. And I would like you to review the whole thing in your mind. And keep breathing. Keep breathing. And now, open your eyes.

End – Emotional Stress Release

Bill: (Opens eyes)

Anny: Anything you want to share with me?

Bill: I think I have a real sense of gratitude, to the people who have been in my life from that time forward. And,

Anny: What created that?

Bill: Um, maybe I just have a lot of room to grow there, appreciate, and really it may have been a life altering, body altering kind of experience. Certainly a lot of good has come into my life since then.

Anny: So where did you get the idea to have to go through that?

Bill: To what?

Anny: Where did you get the idea to have to go through that, to realize all the good things of life?

That is what I am after. I want you to realize that. And it will come to you.

Bill: Oh yah.

Anny: Mm-hmm. Yah, so take a deep breath, and as you exhale, go back to the younger Bill in the hospital, and ask him. By totally recovering, are you still going to have lots of gratitude? And totally, totally trust whatever comes to you. And remember, it is him then, that is going to answer.

Bill: Yah, sure.

Anny: So it is okay to totally recover from head to toe?

Bill: Absolutely.

Anny: Thank him for that. As something inside of you is shifting, and much more is going to come to you, much, much more is going to come to you, and when your subconscious mind gets that message clearly, only then will you be able to open your eyes.

Bill: (Opens eyes)

Anny: So now, you share with me the answer, only if you want to. When you are with those people who had been burned, and the motto was, '*we're not victims, we are survivors*', I would like you to go back there, and with what you know now, what would you tell them?

Bill: I guess I would, just add to the motto, say, "*we are not only survivors, but we are also thrivers!*"

Anny: Bill, what did you volunteer for? The thing is, your subconscious mind finds the path of least resistance. That is true. Go back to how things were before, and you will understand what I am saying. Therefore, when you want something, make sure that the picture in your mind is clear. You understand what I am saying huh?

Bill: Mm-hmm.

Anny: And that realization brings a smile on your face, let me tell you! You say, *oh, do not tell me,* like everybody else!
Bill: It's a, pretty severe way to get out of a bad marriage, is it not?

Anny: Ya. Absolutely! And very acceptable too!

Bill: Man! (laughing)

Anny: And very acceptable too, right? Everybody understands, and everybody is – hey! (laughing) So,

Bill: I got out! (laughing)

Anny: And you did not think of that before, did you?
Yah, (laughing) now, let us completely fix this, if you want to.

Bill: Yes, let us do it.

Anny: When you think, each time you think about what happened with that fire, where do you see it? Where is it sitting in your vision? As you are figuring it out I am getting the target. Where is it in your vision? Each time you see it in your vision? Where does it sit, each time you talk about it, where is it sitting, in your vision?

Bill: I have to look for it, I cannot find it all over.

Anny: All over, huh?

Bill: No I have to look for it, I cannot even find it right now.

Anny: Okay, well talk to me about it, and I will look. Do you remember, can you give me a description of that table? How did that table look like?

Bill: Yah, that is just what I was looking for right now, well it had the fondue on it. It was a wooden table, a big wooden table, a big heavy table. And it had plates on it, but it was in flames, big high ones.

Anny: Where were the children sitting?

Bill: They were behind the table with me.

Anny: But where? On the front, left, right, both sides?

Bill: On both sides of me.

Anny: On both sides. Okay, for whatever reason you keep looking at me there, (his right-hand center vision),

Bill: Yah, that is-

Anny: There. So there is something about it, there.
Okay so I am going to decide that, because I noticed that before.
Each time that you saw it there, so there was something about it that is anchored, and from what I understand, I know what it is, which modality.
I do not know what it is, but I know which modality. Okay.

Eye Movement Integration

Bill: It is a long time ago, Anny.

Anny: Ya.

Bill And,

Anny: You see, you are there again.

Bill I do not think of it that often, and I almost have to pull it up and put it back on file.

Anny: Okay. Alright. Okay. So, when you think about it, we are going to count. Okay, I need a number, because we are going to gauge if it goes higher or lower, or whatever.

Bill Okay.

Anny: Well, it is 100. We have to start somewhere, ok. 100. And now, how do you – the moment you are thinking about it, what comes to your mind?

The first thing that comes to your mind.

Bill: Um, what I need to do?

Anny: No, the first thing that comes, what is it?

Bill: Protect my children.

Anny: Okay, but so it is a thought, a picture, a sound, or? Or a feeling, or?

Bill: No, it is actually an image.

Anny: An image.

Bill: Running, running out of the house.

Anny: Okay an image.
An image. Alright, very good. Okay so I am going to ask you to follow my target here, and tell me how it is going? And you tell me also if you prefer me to be a little further back or closer to you?

(targeting across top and left-hand side)

Bill: Nothing, it was just faded, it does not feel any different.

Anny: Okay, is it clearer now, or dimmer, or - ?

Bill: Just the same.

Anny: It is the same, Okay.

So*, (targeting triangularly across top, to bottom center)*

Keep your gaze here. Keep your gaze on my target.

(circling the top left hand corner) How is it now?

Bill: A little bit of a body intensity.

Anny: Okay, a body intensity. So, coming from 100, what is it then?

Bill: Maybe 120.

Anny: 120. Okay. Very good. Alright.

(targeting triangularly across top to center right hand side)

Anny: So now? Now?

Bill: It is about the same intensity, but it is more, I actually heard sound this time.

Anny: Which?

Bill: I heard sound this time.

Anny: Can you tell me what were the sounds?

Bill: People's voices.

Anny: People's voices?
Bill: Mm-hmm, people's voices, my step on the hardwood floor, um - clatter of some sort. Flames.

Anny: Okay, how do you feel about that?

Bill: Well I never visualized it and had sound before.

Anny: Mm-hmm. Okay.

Bill: And I have visualized it and felt it, but never had the sound before.

Anny: Of course, never had the sound. Is it not that interesting? Okay. So now, always keep your gaze, and would you prefer me to go a little further, or it does not matter? Okay.

(targeting top to bottom – diamond shape)

How is it now?

Bill: Ah, about 90.

Anny: Good. Now, I am going to check another point that we did not. And then keep it for the last.

(targeting diagonally from left to right upper to lower corners)

How is it?

Bill: That just stirred me right up again.

Anny: That is the emotion. That is where it is. ***(right hand, center)***

Bill: Ya.

Anny: That is the point of emotions.

Bill: More in my chest.
Anny: So now, how about clearing that?

Bill: Sure.

Anny: Because you were here, it was also that that was a major one. The emotions. And whatever you feel like doing now, understand that it is when he got in that accident, that felt, he felt the way you feel now. So whatever is the emotion, allow it. Allow it.

So close your eyes for a moment, and allow that emotion. Allow it. It was Bill then, that did not express an emotion. And then open your eyes. Surprised you huh?

Bill: Ya, for sure

Anny: It is the emotion, that is all.
So let us clear that, so that just like on the chart there, it is gone. Okay?

Bill: Sure.

Anny: Alright.

(targeting across the top diagonally to across bottom, diagonally again to top)

How is it now?

Bill: I still have some emotion left there, but it is a different kind of emotion, it is more like a relief.

Anny: It is a relief emotion? Okay. So what is the number?

Bill: Well actually, it felt kind of good, so I would actually have to give it a plus number.

Anny: Okay, now I would like you to go inside of you, and decide which way will be the best to really, really see what you did, now?
Bill: The last one.

Anny: The last one, okay, my intuition said check *one thing*, and then we will do the last one. Okay, my intuition said, so I am going to follow my intuition, and then I will do what you said, okay?

(targeting in a full square, circling the center left hand side)

What is happening here?

Bill: It is stirring me up again.

Anny: What?

Bill: Stirring me up again.

Anny: Ya, the sound? It is the sound. That has how come my intuition said, "no, no, no."

Bill: It is here.

Anny: Okay. So it is not a surprise. So, what is the number again?

Bill: If we started at 100, I would say 40. Uh-huh.

Anny: Alright. Something more with the sound, huh. Okay, let us fix that, and then we will go to dessert. Okay? Alright.

Bill: Not much of anything.

Anny: What?

Bill: Not much of anything.

Anny: Zero?

Bill: Ya,

Anny: Okay, so, ah what did I do here, I did like this. Okay so now we are going to check it out again. Okay.

(targeting in a full square)

What is happening now?

Bill: It is fixed.

Anny: It is fixed. How does that feel?

Bill: It is fine. It is fine.

Anny: And how does it feel that it is fine?

Bill: It is good. Whatever is left there, is if anything, positive energy, if anything.

Anny: Okay.

Bill: Ya.

Anny: So how do you feel about that?

Bill: Well that is fine, that is great. That is better than some of those anxious kinds of feelings.

End of eye movement integration
and
collapsing all anchors.

Anny: Okay, take a slow, deep breath now, and as you exhale, close your eyes.

That is right. And find yourself in front **of** Bill who is very much aware of the way of his marriage.
Just give him some sign of encouragement, whatever is acceptable to him, so that you know that he knows you know all about it now, and you feel fine with it all, and most of all that you understand him very well.

And with a smile, make him realize that, you know, things could have been much smoother than that. So make him aware of a few things there, and having a good sense of humour helps a lot.

So, say, man, are not we clever! Explain to him what was resolved and dissolved, and that it is fine. That to your amazement, you are discovering that things will be better than before.

As something inside of you has shifted. I do not know what has shifted. And you do not know what has shifted. All that I know is that very deep inside of you something has shifted. And how that awareness is powerful.

It is bringing everything better than before, so that all this or something even better, now manifests itself in your attitude, your behavior, your life, in a most delightful way, and the benefits of this session, and the benefit of all the counseling you had prior to this session, will stay with you for hours, days, weeks, months, and years to come, much to your surprise and delight.

And bless your family, bless your friends, bless your pets if you have any, and that includes your pet projects! Bless your possessions, bless your wishes, bless and thank, from the bottom of your heart, the younger Bills that came to you today and were honest and candid enough to allow you to resolve all this.

Bless that light of yours, that very beautiful light of yours, that mini sun in your chest, and thank God, whoever you perceive God to be, for the wonders of life.

You are more relaxed than you have been for a while and each time you enter this type of relaxation you will enjoy a deeper and much, much better quality of relaxation. And so it is. And so it is.

So now, I am going to count from 1 to 5 and then I will say, your eyes are open and you are fully aware. You are rested, refreshed, relaxed, renewed, at peace with yourself and with the world around you.

One, slowly, calmly, easily, and gently, returning to full awareness once again, enjoying a sharp mind, a clear head, and a tranquil heart.

Two, each muscle and nerve in your body is loose, limp, and relaxed, and you feel wonderfully good, enjoying a sharp mind, a clear head, and a tranquil heart.

Three, from head to toe you are feeling better in every way; physically better, mentally better, emotionally cool, calm, and serene, enjoying a sharp mind, a clear head, and a tranquil heart.

Four, your eyes begin to feel sparkling clear, as though they were bathed in cool spring water, and only when everything is set and accepted within you, only then will you be able to open your eyes.

Although I say five now, you will only be able to open your eyes when everything has been accepted.

Bill: (Eyes open)

Anny: What surprised you?
Bill: I know that I have done a lot better than some of the other survivors, just really crashed, their lives go absolutely all terrible. And what surprised me is how come I had to do that? That is what shocked me. And that is nuts.

Anny: Hmm?

Bill: That is nuts. Just to go through that kind of an episode just to get out of a bad relationship. Come on! You know, just slip out the back, Jack. Make a new plan, Stan. Do not go toast yourself. Just dessert!

Anny: No, that is the way it is.

Bill: Ya, and quite frankly I forgive myself for that. That is who I was at the time and that is what I did. That is who I was then, that is what I had to work with. That is what I did. That is that. (laughing)

Anny: Now you know, when I say from day one, there is no victims, there is only volunteers. And it is incredible what we do with ourselves because we do not have a better way. And your subconscious mind will find a way, let me tell you.

Bill: There is another side benefit from it.

Anny: Of course there is!

Bill: And uh, and you know, like sitting here right now, uh I had no animosity toward my spouse, that was the truth, I cannot blame her; I did not.

Anny: So what have you learned?

Bill: Well you know, if you want out of something just say so.

Anny: Right!

Bill: Just say so.

Anny: Just say so.

Bill: Hey, instead of agonizing or trying to go crazy and nuts to make something work.

Anny: Do you think I can have a hug? (laughing) And thank you for being such a good volunteer.

Bill: Okay.

Questions About Past Life Regression Practice

- Question 1 -
- Question 2 -
- Question 3 -
- Question 4 -
- Question 5 -

Past Life Regression Practice

First remember, the client knows everything, the therapist knows nothing. It helps keeping our ego in check….

Since we go from effect back to cause, when in need of help a client will spontaneously go to where they are supposed to go. When a client goes spontaneously into a past life, we only use our skills to help them resolve whatever has to be resolved.

However, a client will sometimes ask for a past life session. The following exercise will make it easy for you to lead a client into another time in another life.

For the training, let us keep it light and very beneficial to you. And please note you can read the instructions if you wish to do so. It works!

Instructions for the client

Is there something you love to do and wish you could do it better and sustain it?
It could be drawing, singing, gardening, building, healing, teaching, whatever you really like to do. Chose something "light!"

Ask the client to have that skill in mind as the facilitator will lead you into a trance and a fascinating voyage.

Instructions for the facilitator

Using your favorite induction, lead the client into a very pleasant state of relaxation.

The prayer:

… as I am asking for your protection and your well being and I say "God, please allow only good things to come to us, and for this blessing we give thanks."

And now you ask to be placed into the protection of your very own light, your very own light, your spark of life. It is like a mini sun in your chest. Some people can see it. Some people can feel it. Some people simply know it is there. That light of yours. The beautiful light of yours. Let it shine. Let it shine. Let it shine throughout every cell of your body. Throughout your aura. Cleansing your body. Cleansing your aura. Strengthening your body. Strengthening your aura. Extending itself at one arm's length above you, beneath you, at each side of you, in front of you and behind you and mentally repeat with me "This is my body. This is my space. Only light can come to me. Only light can come from me. Only my light can be here."

And as you take a slow deep breath and exhale, find yourself in your home in the room you like the most to be in and as you are there, standing there, become aware of your light, your spark of life. And as you take a slow deep breath and exhale, extend it to the property line, under the basement and over the tallest tree or building on your property and give that light of yours a job. You want that property to be healthy, safe and most enjoyable and whatever else you want. Give your light a job. Give your light a job. And then as you take a slow deep breath and exhale, allow yourself to go to the right level of relaxation for the work at hand.

Suggestions for the session.

When you are relaxed, your subconscious mind is open and receptive to the suggestion you are receiving now.

And during this session, the sound of my voice will make you go deeper and deeper into relaxation.

During this session, each time I touch your knee (Anchoring deepening the trance) you will go deeper and deeper into relaxation, and ***during this session***, the familiar sounds in this room will make you go deeper and deeper into relaxation. Your subconscious mind, is open and receptive to the suggestions you are receiving now, and will sort all things out, revealing to you whatever you want to know and understand.

The information will come to you clearly and in a way that you will remember and understand, much to you surprise and delight.

Slowly inhale and as you slowly exhale, sleep now. Inhale. Slowly exhale. Sleep now. When I say sleep now, this is not the sleep you experience when you fall asleep at night. I am talking about hypnotic sleep. This means that you relax completely your mind and your body. Your subconscious mind, freed of all restraint, is open and receptive to the suggestions you are receiving during this session.

And during this experience, the sound of my voice makes you so relaxed, so comfortable.

Also during this experience, the familiar sounds of the room will make you more and more relaxed. More and more at peace. Let all your cares fade away. Fade away. Fade away. Fade away.

And now, as you take a slow deep breath and exhale, your subconscious mind is open and very receptive to the suggestions you are receiving now, It will sort all things out and reveal to you whatever it feels you should know and understand about the question and your reason to go into a trance right now.

And I am asking your subconscious mind to reveal it to you at most unexpected time. It will always be very comforting. The information will be quite delightful.
And for this blessing, we give thanks.

And now, as you are listening to my voice, going deeper and deeper into that very special quality of relaxation, find yourself at the top of a very beautiful set of stairs. Beautiful. It could be indoors; it could be outdoors. A beautiful set of stairs.

And as you are standing there, at the top of this beautiful staircase let your quest come to your awareness. Whatever you wanted to accomplish as you are entering this exercise is coming back to mind.

And as you are there, look around you. Close to you there is a table with loose sheets of paper, pens of different colours of ink and a chair.

In your mind, walk to the table, sit down, take a sheet of paper and notice the colour of ink of the pen you are choosing.

And write down your quest, your reason to go into another time in another life. What do you enjoy doing and want to be better at, or learn to enjoy doing. There is something that you want to know. Something that you want to experience and sustain. Write it down.

Facilitator: write it down too as you voice it.

And now, in your mind, get up, put down the pen and pick up the sheet of paper with your quest written on it.
And find yourself at the top of that beautiful set of stairs. Look around you. It is beautiful and safe and comfortable to be there.

And you have one hand on the railing.
That is right.

Notice the feel of the railing under your hand.
That is right, holding the piece of paper in the other hand.

And notice how you feel deep inside, as you are there standing at the top of the most beautiful set of stairs. And read what you wrote on the sheet of paper you are holding in your hand. FACILITATOR, read it out loud.

And as you are contemplating your quest, start going down the stairs one step at a time, telling yourself that with each step down, you are going deeper and deeper into relaxation. Feel the railing under your hand, the sheet of paper in the other hand, the steps under your feet, telling yourself that with each step down, you go deeper and deeper into a special quality of relaxation. Deeper and deeper. Deeper and deeper.

And now, as you start to go down the stairs one step at a time, you feel yourself going deeper and deeper in a very beautiful experience of relaxation. Very pleasant, very beautiful experience of relaxation.

Going down the steps one step at a time.

That is right.
Feel the steps under your feet. Feel the steps as you are going down the stairs one step at a time.

That is right.
One step at a time. That is right. One step at a time. One step at a time. One step at a time.

And when you are at the bottom of the stairs, sit on the last step and you read what you wrote on that piece of paper.

FACILITATOR, read it out loud.

And as you are sitting there on the last step, you notice a blackboard in front of you and close by, a door, a door to a very special place.

In your mind, you get up and walk to the blackboard, pick up a chalk and write on the blackboard the numbers from ten down to one. And when you are done, simply nod.

Put the chalk down, pick up the eraser and slowly, one by one, erase the numbers starting with the number 10, telling yourself that with each number down, you are going deeper and deeper into relaxation. And when you are done, simply nod.

And now, becoming more and more relaxed, holding that piece of paper in one hand, walk towards the door. The door to another time, another life.

And when you are there, touch the door. Feel the door. Notice the details of the door and know that the door is going to open into another time, another life, a life when you were very good at what you like to do, and truly enjoy it.
And read what you wrote on that sheet of paper, The what-for of this experience.

FACILITATOR, read it out loud.

So now as you are taking a slow deep breath and as you exhale, open the door. Does it make a sound? Pass through the door. Close the door behind you and turn around.

You will find that there is a mirror there. You could call it a magic mirror.

There was a reason for you to go into this trance. Remember your question. What awareness do you want to have? What do you want to learn?

What do you want to know? And now become very much aware of how you feel as you walk towards that very, very special mirror.

And now as you are standing now in front of what one could call the magic mirror, look into it and realize that the mirror is, in fact, a door to another time, another life, when you experienced the expertise you want now. A time when you enjoyed so much what you enjoy doing now, and you want that expertise again, and you want it now.

Be there. Be there! Find yourself back into that life. Enjoy the experience. Be there.

Enjoy it and most of all, trust the awareness that is coming to you.
Trust the experience.
Welcome the events.

Facilitator, please allow your client to experience discovering how good they were at what they still enjoy doing and make them talk about what is going on so it is recorded. Ask what was the highlight of that life.

Ask client to read again what is written on the peace of paper. And voiced it too.

Remember it is important to make your client go though the dead experience, and observe where the other self is going.

As you are observing where the one in the past life is going, you will then know if, for whatever reason, an other entity has showed up, instead of the client's own self.

At this point into the training, just act as this is normal and proceed with the session.

And now as you have experienced and enjoyed the answer to your quest, from the depth of your being, you remember clearly the recommendations of that part of you in another time, another life.

And now, turn around and walk towards the door. As you are about to open the door to leave the room, turn around and look at the "Magic Mirror". You know that more and more information will come to you as the days are going by, remembering clearly the experience and feeling at peace with yourself and with the world around you.

As you take a slow deep breath, and exhale, open the door. Does it make a sound? Pass through the door, close the door behind you and find yourself at the bottom of the staircase that brought you to this journey.

With one hand on the railing, holding the piece of paper in the other hand, slowly come back up the stairs, one step at the time, telling yourself that with each step up, you are coming back to full awareness, remembering your experience, remembering the recommendations.

And when you are back at the top of the staircase, slowly walk towards the table, sit in the chair and read the quest you wrote on the piece of paper, feeling relaxed and at peace, having learned something important to you, knowing more information will come to you.

Coming back to now

And now I am going to count from 1 to 5 and I will say:
Your eyes are open.
You are fully aware.
Feeling refreshed, relaxed, renewed.
Totally, totally at peace with yourself and with the world around you.

One, slowly, calmly, easy, gently, beginning to return to full awareness once again. Enjoying a sharp mind, a clear head and a tranquil heart.

Two, each muscle and nerve in your body is loose, limp, relaxed and you feel wonderfully good.
You feel at peace with yourself and with the world around you.
Enjoying a sharp mind, a clear head and a tranquil heart.

Three, from head to toe you are feeling so much better in every way.
Physically better. Mentally better. Emotionally cool, calm and serene.
Enjoying a sharp mind, a clear head and a tranquil heart.

Four, your eyes begin to feel sparkling clear as bathed in cool spring water.

Five, eyelids open. Open your eyes. You are fully aware. Take a slow deep breath. Open your eyes and give yourself a very good stretch.

Suggestion to the facilitator

It is important that you trust your intuition and use deepening techniques should you realise the client is not staying in a trance.

Please note: as your client is experiencing what they perceive, make the client talk about their experience, only asking open ended questions. For example: when we ask "are you a man or a woman?" without realising it, our voice is suggesting the choice. If necessary, ask "what is your gender?" make them explain what they are experiencing, asking "and what happen then", "how do you feel", use your own judgement about it.

Help your client the way you would help them when they spontaneously go into a past life.

What is written here is simply a guideline to give you an idea of what you can do to lead a person into a past life. At this point into the training, you know hypnosis well. Simply trust your ability to help your client. Remember: it is their story, it is their truth and honour it.

At the end of the session, ask

"What surprised you?

"What have you learned? Do you feel comfortable telling me about it?

Students have some incredibly beautiful experiences. Choose something "light" and you will most likely experience an enjoyable and enlightening experience too.

I love you all,

Anny Slegten

Questions About Dual Past Life Regression Practice

- Question 1 -

- Question 2 -

- Question 3 -

- Question 4 -

- Question 5 -

Dual Regression

This is a technique I learned from William Baldwin, D.D.S., Ph.D.
The following is an exert from the class manual:
Regression Therapy, Spirit Releasement Therapy

Tracing a relationship together can be a romantic excursion in time for two people. Dual regression can be a wonderful addition to couples counselling although it is not limited to romantic relationships. The induction consists of a chakra linkage through visualization of light color energy. The two people lie side by side on a bed, on the floor or in adjacent reclining chairs. Questions are directed at each of participants separately. Each person remains in his or her own experience and answers appropriately, even though each can hear the others answers.

Once the two people are comfortable, side by side but not touching, the therapist guides the induction.

Therapist: "Close your eyes and focus inward. Focus deep inside to the very center of your being. Find your own spark of light there, your own light. Deep inside. Feel it. See it. Sense it there. Imagine it there. Deep inside you. Imagine that the spark of light glows warmly and expands in every direction. Upward and downward. The light expands clear into the tips of your toes to the top of your head. From fingertip to fingertip. Filling every cell of your body. Imagine the light expanding outward. Beyond the boundaries of your body about an arm's length in every direction. A shimmering bubble of golden white light all around you." The invocation of light is important in any altered state experience.

Therapist: "Imagine now at the base of your spine, the location of the first chakra, the color of red. Bright, clear, apple red. The base chakra, the energy of survival. Sense that color red flowing upward and outward, arching across toward your partner, connecting with the first chakra of your partner. Visualize an arch of red connecting your base chakra to the base chakra of your partner."

Therapist: "Imagine now at the level of your genitals, the second chakra, the color orange. Bright, clear, tangerine orange. The energy of generativity and sexuality. Sense that color orange arching across toward your partner connecting with the second chakra. An arch of orange and an arch of red, connecting the two of you."

Therapist: "Imagine now at your solar plexus the color yellow. Bright, clear, lemon yellow. The third chakra, the energy of intellect, power, control. Sense that color yellow arching across toward your partner, connecting with the third chakra. An arch of orange, an arch of red and an arch of yellow, connecting the two of you."

Therapist: "Imagine now at the level of your heart the color green. Bright, clear, emerald green. The heart chakra, the energy of unconditional love. Sense that color green arching across toward your partner, connecting with the heart chakra, the fourth chakra.

An arch of orange, an arch of red, an arch of yellow and an arch of green connecting the two of you."

Therapist: "Imagine now at the level of your throat the color blue. Deep, clear, blue. The throat chakra, the energy of creativity and communication. Sense that color blue arching across toward your partner, connecting with the throat chakra. The fifth chakra. An arch of orange, an arch of red, an arch of yellow, an arch of green and an arch of blue connecting the two of you."

Therapist: "Imagine now at the level of your brow the color violet. Deep, clear, soothing violet. The brow chakra. The seat of intuition, the third eye. Sense that violet color arching across toward your partner, connecting with the sixth chakra, the brow chakra. An arch of red, an arch of orange, an arch of yellow, an arch of green, an arch of blue and an arch of violet connecting the two of you."

Therapist: "Imagine now at the top of your head the white light. Bright, clear, white light, the combination of all colors. The crown chakra, the energy of the highest consciousness. Sense that white light flowing from you. Surrounding you and your partner. The arches of red, orange, yellow, green and blue connecting the two of you and engulfed in white light."

Therapist: "Imagine yourself lifting out of your body, out through the white light, together in spirit with your partner. Back now, back in time now. Back together to another time and place when you knew each other. Allow the light to carry you back into the experience of another lifetime when you knew each other. Locate another lifetime when you knew each other and you interacted together. Find yourself in the experience of another lifetime.
(pause).

Therapist: "What is the first thing you experience? What is the first thing you are aware of in this place?"

These instructions are given slowly and clearly in a soft voice. Whichever person speaks first the therapist responds and pursues the conversation for a few minutes. At a logical stopping place the therapist switches to the other partner.

Therapist: "As she is experiencing ____________________, what are you experiencing?"

The other partner may be in the same moment, at an earlier time or later time in the same lifetime, or in another lifetime. The conversation is pursued briefly, then the focus switches on the first partner.

Therapist: "As he is experiencing ____________________, what is happening to you? What are you aware of?"

If the partners are involved in the same experience it is easier to continue. If they are clearly not connecting yet at an appropriate time, not in the midst of a trauma but in a more neutral scene, the therapist urges them to locate a mutual experience.

Therapist: "Move forward or backward in time in the lifetime you are experiencing. Locate the very first time you are together. Locate the first time your recognize each other. Locate the very first experience together." (pause) "What are you experiencing?" This may lead them to their first meeting, however unusual it may be.

In a class setting, two therapists Al and Bill, choose to explore what past connections they might share. The student therapist was nervous about the process, doubting her ability. Al described living alone in a small hut, far from the town. He was a soldier and received an urgent summons. The town was under siege.

Bill was a scholar in a cloistered setting, living a sheltered life behind the walls of the sanctuary. The soldier was part of a group sent to protect the sanctuary, an important part of this town. The attackers were turned away but the soldier was mortally wounded.

After the battle had subsided, several of the scholars went out of the building to where the wounded soldiers lay. Bill carried the dying soldier Al into the walled enclosure where the wounded could be tended. Al died before anything could be done. He had literally given his life in defence of the scholars and their sanctuary.

The student therapist could not make sense of the experiences being related until about halfway through the session when the soldier described the sanctuary walls form the outside. It seemed like the outside of the same building the scholar described from the inside. The connection between these two friends came with the death of the soldier.

They both understood the profound nature of the unconditional love expressed in the scene. For the soldier doing his duty, it was the giving of his life for unknown persons inside. For the cloistered scholar who dedicated his life to education of his students, it was the realization that someone had died to protect the sanctuary and preserve his life and purpose.

PLEASE REMEMBER TO DIS-ENGAGE SO BOTH PARTIES ARE SET FREE FROM EACH OTHER AND ARE BACK TO PRESENT TIME.

To disengage after been connected though the chakras, make both parties simultaneously go through each chakra to disconnect, starting by the crown chakra.

- Now, become aware of the arch of white light at the top of your head and disconnect yourself from your partner, recalling your energy.

- Going down to the brow chakra, notice the beautiful violet colour of the arch. Recall your arch; disconnect yourself from your partner.

- The blue colour of your throat chakra, Disconnect.

- Now, become aware of the arch that connects you through the heart chakra. Bright, clear, emerald green. Retract your arch. Set your partner free.

- As you move down at your yellow solar plexus. Reclaim your energy. Disconnect.

- Down to the chakra just below the navel. The base chakra. It is orange in colour. Disconnect, recall that arch.

- And now, at the base of your spine is the root chakra. The chakra you sit on. Bright red. Take a deep breath, and as you exhale disconnect completely, setting you both free, back into your body claiming your own space.

Sometimes, to help disconnecting or feeling the disconnection is not completed, I pass my hand up and down between the two persons with the intention of cutting the energy cords.

Why is it so important to disconnect both parties?

There is a very deep bonding when one connects with the chakras. Therefore, it is important to disconnect after going into a past life with someone for the simple reason the bonding is inappropriate at this point in time. I witnessed this during my training with Bill Baldwin. The agony of that couple was very noticeable since, in this life, been connected that way was totally inappropriate.

Because the intent is to go into a past life experienced together, connecting through the chakras is connecting at soul level. It is a deep ether connection that transports you trough time and space and evokes sentiments and feelings from another time.

In other words, the intent is what counts as we connect through the chakras.

<u>If the intent is to visit or experience a connection in a past life</u>, it will align the energy of the persons and act like an emotional magnet in another place in another time.

Couples ask for a dual regression when there seem to be an unsuccessful pattern in their relationship and want to "go to the bottom of it" to understand what is going on between them. They usually have a sense of "It happens again with him/her" or "we are doing it again". I have some extremely very funny stories about that!

<u>If the intent is for an experience in the now</u>, it will align the energy of the persons and act like an emotional magnet.

The best way to understand the magnetic power of this method is to connect that way, with your spouse of course, and you will experience the results of this method of deep bonding.

It also works very well by telepathy!

After learning about this and listening to the information I give in class, one of the students, whose husband is rather lazy in bed, connected their chakras by telepathy. The results were interesting.

That morning, arriving late to class, beaming, the student explained that, to check this out, she connected her husband's and her chakras by telepathy. During breakfast and after showering, getting dressed and ready to come for class, her husband was still in the kitchen, waiting for her and very aroused said "Do you have time?", something he never did before....

Anny

Hypnotist Code of Ethics

I commit myself to conduct my professional relationships in accordance with this Code of Ethics and subscribe to the following statements:

1. I regard as my primary professional obligation the welfare of my client, whether individual or group.

2. I will comply with the requirements of the law in the jurisdiction where I practice. I will not discriminate against any person, group, or class on the basis of race, ethnicity, national origin, color, sex, sexual orientation, gender identity or expression, age, marital status, political belief, religion, immigration status, or mental or physical ability.

3. I will offer services only within my scope of practice and the boundaries of competence, and the recognized knowledge and competences of the profession of hypnotherapy, including supervision and consultation, whether in person or remotely.

4. I will not claim to diagnose, prescribe treatment for, or treat any mental or physical illness unless I possess qualifications, certification and/or licensure additional to hypnotherapy certification, which legally entitles me to do so in the jurisdiction where I practice.

5. I will not use any licensed or restricted title or other professional designation to which I am not legally entitled in the jurisdiction where I practice.

6. I will advise a client whose requirements are outside my boundaries of competence to seek an appropriate alternative service.

7. I will advise any client presenting symptoms of physical illness, including pain, to seek the advice of a medical practitioner if this has not already been obtained.

8. I will not guarantee cures for any condition or make misleading claims or statements as to the outcome of the services I offer, in any form of advertising, verbally, in print or digital promotions. I will be socially responsible and adhere to the rules of "truth-in-advertising" in the marketing statements I make. These will be legal, accurate and fair. I will avoid the use of superlatives, misleading information, and deceptive claims.

9. I will make clear to the client, prior to the provision of services, the terms, conditions, and charges for my services.

10. I will keep confidential any information obtained in the course of service within the legal limits of reporting requirements in the jurisdiction where I practice. I will disclose any such limits of confidentiality to my clients prior to providing services. I will ensure that the client's anonymity and privacy is safeguarded in the publication of any clinical material.

11. I will do my best to ensure secure technology and will disclose to clients in the event of a breach. I will discuss with clients, students and/or those I mentor my policies concerning the use of technology in the provision of professional services. I will obtain informed consent before making audio or video recordings or permitting observation of services to clients by a third party. When using technology to deliver services, I will ensure I have the necessary knowledge and skills to provide such services in a competent manner. This includes an understanding of the special communication challenges when using technology and the ability to implement strategies to address these challenges.

12. I will obtain the written consent of a parent or guardian before providing services to a minor.

13. I will not sexually harass or make sexual advances, solicitation, requests for sexual favors or any other verbal, written, electronic or attempt any physical contact of a sexual nature with any client, supervisee, student, or colleague. I will not engage in intimate social contact with a client until a period of at least two years from the conclusion of therapeutic work with that client.

14. I will undertake continuing professional development and education.

15. I accept responsibility to help protect the community against unethical practice by any individual engaged in providing hypnotherapy services e.g. by reporting professional misconduct to the proper bodies or authorities, including unethical conduct using technology.

16. I will treat with respect the findings, views and actions of professional colleagues and use appropriate channels to express my opinions on these matters. I will avoid unwarranted negative criticism of colleagues in verbal, written, and electronic communications with clients or with other professionals.

17. I will conduct myself in a manner consistent with upholding the good reputation of the profession of hypnotherapy.

18. I will distinguish clearly in public between my statements and actions as an individual and as a representative of an organization.

19. I will not engage in any dual or multiple relationships with students or clients that cause harm or exploitation. I understand I am responsible for setting clear, appropriate, and culturally sensitive boundaries, and terms of contracts need to be made clear at the outset and maintained during any Dual Relationships. Dual relationships or Multiple Relationships refer to any situation where multiple roles exist between a therapist and a client. Examples of dual relationships are when the client is also a student, friend, family member, employee or business associate of the therapist.

20. I will take reasonable steps to ensure that documentation in electronic and/or paper records is accurate and reflects the services provided. I will transfer or dispose of clients' records in a manner that protects clients' confidentiality and is consistent with applicable laws governing records.

I understand that the maintenance of high ethical standards is an important support to the professional standing of all Hypnotherapists.

I agree to conduct my practice and all professional interactions in strict accordance with rules and regulations in effect now or in the future.

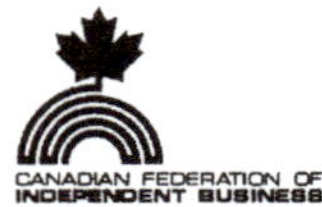

Privacy Legislation

Compliance guidelines for your business

M-IN0121-0312(213)

Does this apply to me?.... *YES!*

The federal ***Personal Information Protection and Electronic Documents Act***, comes into effect on January 1, 2004. As a result, ***all*** businesses are subject to new stringent guidelines regarding the collection, storage and disclosure of private and personal information collected on individuals. Failure to comply with the Act can result in lawsuits and the awarding of punitive damages.

Businesses located in Quebec are already regulated under provincial privacy legislation (for information on Quebec's legislation go to the website for *La Commission d'accès à l'information du Québec* **http://www.cai.gouv.qc.ca/**).

The following is a brief outline of how the privacy legislation affects your business:

WHAT IS PERSONAL INFORMATION?

The Privacy legislation defines personal information as: age, name, weight, height, medical records, ID numbers, income, ethnic origin, blood type, opinions, evaluations, comments, social status, employee files, disciplinary action, credit records, loan records, existence of a dispute between a consumer and a merchant and intentions (for example, to acquire goods or services, or change jobs.)

WHAT THE ACT COVERS

Accountability: The Act states that organizations must have a documented Privacy policy, and appoint an internal Privacy Expert/Commissioner who is knowledgeable about the legislation and able to train persons who will be collecting, using, or disclosing personal information.

Identification of Purposes: Individuals must be informed of the purpose for the collection, and how the information might be used or disclosed to other outside organizations.

Consent: There are three types of consent that can be used, A. Express Consent/Permission (Opt-in), B. Negative Option (Opt-out), and C. Implied Consent. Information of a more sensitive nature (health, medical, financial) will require stronger methods of obtaining consent (*Please refer to the Privacy Commissioner web site for a detailed description of these options.)*

Limiting Collection: Gather only the information that is necessary for the identified purposes.

Limit Use, Disclosure, and Retention: Personal information must only be used for the purposes for which consent has been given. Only keep the information for as long as it is necessary.

Accuracy: Personal Information should be accurate. Processes/procedures must be put in place for persons to flag and rectify inaccuracies in their own personal information.

Safeguards: Measures must be taken to ensure that personal information is secured, such as locked cabinets, electronic firewalls, and limited staff access.

Openness: Privacy policies and practices should be available in a public document or web site.

Individual Access: Ability to inform individuals how their information was collected, used and disclosed, including a list of with whom their information has been shared.

Provide Recourse: Privacy policies should describe complaint resolution procedures.

Recycled Paper

Transcript: A Way To Ground Ourselves

So here you are, listening to this relaxing and grounding recording, very relaxing, very, very pleasant.

And, as you are there, find yourself outside. Somewhere where you would like a tree to grow. Yes, you would love to have a tree there to grow.

(Pause)

So, as you are there, in your mind, imagine yourself, being a seed, the seed of a tree, that is right, the seed of a tree. A tree you love, something that makes you feel great when you see that tree, you feel strong, healthy, and surprisingly good looking.

So here you are. You are a seed, the seed of a beautiful tree, and as you are there, you discover it is a perfect place for the seed to germinate, and you can feel the seed swelling, so to speak, and starting to establish itself, starting to establish itself, into the earth.

And, as the seed is really starting to establish itself, and you know, claim its dominion, so to speak, you can feel, a stem coming out, you can feel it. And, the ground is fertile, and the weather is perfect to keep the ground moist and the weather is nice and warm. The perfect temperature for that particular tree.

And as you are there, in your mind, you are the tree. And you can feel the trunk starting to get taller and taller, and stronger. As the tree is getting taller and stronger, you can feel the roots firmly establishing themselves into the ground, really. The perfect roots for the type of tree you are.

And as you are there, you notice that, as the tree is getting taller, and claiming dominion over the earth, really establishing itself, you realise the resilience of that tree. As the wind may make it sway sometimes, and as it is growing, more and more mature, notice how more and more resilient it is. So that when the weather is not as appropriate as it should be, it grows very well anyway.

Yes. The tree sometimes does not grow that fast, because the weather may not be appropriate, and then as soon as the weather and moisture is appropriate it catches up.

As it is growing, growing, growing, and the roots are going deeper and deeper and wider and wider into the earth, claiming dominion over its space. You can feel that tree growing, the trunk getting stronger and stronger as it gets higher and higher.

That is right, getting stronger and stronger as it is getting higher and higher. And notice how the roots are accommodating the tree so that the tree can really grow. Having beautiful branches and a beautiful shape, so to speak, as the roots are getting deeper and deeper, wider and wider. And the tree, getting taller and taller, become an absolutely beautiful, incredible tree.

And, as you are, there, in your mind, you are that tree. That absolutely incredible, beautiful, healthy tree. With a smile, you realise the deeper the roots, the higher the tree. Yes, the deeper the roots, the higher the tree. A perfect balance. A perfect balance.

That is right. The deeper the roots the higher the tree. And as you have the roots really going deeper and deeper into the earth, the tree is getting higher and higher towards the sky, towards the Universe.

And as you are experiencing that perfect balance, the beautiful balance, you realize, that the more grounded you are, the higher your awareness of what the Universe is all about.

Because of that perfect balance you are solid within this planet as you are reaching the life up above. So breathe in that very pleasant sensation, breathe it in deeply realizing the deeper the roots, the higher the tree.

That is right, the deeper the roots, the higher the tree.

So the more you establish yourself on this planet firmly grounded, appreciating life on this planet, there is that other part of you who is more and more connected to that Universal energy that is more and more comfortable at totally, totally, totally acknowledging the incredible life from up above, feeling comfortable with it, feeling perfect balance with it.

And now when you see a tree you will understand what it represents to you: the deeper the roots the higher the tree, the deeper your understanding of what life is all about on this planet, the higher your understanding, your knowledge, your intuition about that other side of life. And for this blessing we give thanks.

So relax, acknowledge what is life to you, really as you can feel the energy moving up the trunk of the tree, and the roots going down, down into the earth to absorb and be nourished by the planet earth.

There is another part of you, that in the trunk of the tree, is going up, up, up, reaching the Celestial energy that is really high and much taller than the depthless of the roots of that tree.

Acknowledge it.
The roots are feeding from the earth.

The trunk, and all of what is about the ground, is nourished by the Devine and being nourished by the Devine can also bring nourishment to the roots of the tree. Enjoy that realization.

Enjoy your own beauty as a human being. Realizing that the more you have your feet on the ground the higher is your understanding of heaven, so to speak. So relax, just relax and enjoy that understanding. When you observe a tree and you know the more established a tree is, the higher it can grow.

And you can feel within you that light of yours connecting with the Universe as it resides in the physical part of you and so it is, and so it is.

(Pause)

So, I am asking your subconscious mind, to be open and very receptive to the suggestions you are receiving now, to shift whatever has to be shifted, heal whatever has to be healed, improve whatever has to be improved, so that all this or something even better, now manifests itself in your attitude, your behaviour, your life, in a most delightful way. Realizing that the deeper the roots, the firmer you are on this planet, the higher you can allow your mind to go and connect with the universe and whoever you perceive God to be.

And for this blessing, we give thanks.

Anny

Online Store, Contact, And More…

You may contact Anny by visiting any of her websites and scroll down the home page to the contact information.

http://www.annyslegten.com
Anny's private website and online store.

http://www.success-and-more.com
To find the description of the many services offered, and more.

http://www.htialberta.com
The Hypnotism Training Institute of Alberta including descriptions of hypnosis and hypnotherapy courses given.

http://www.reiki-canada.com
About the Reiki Training Centre of Canada.

http://www.slegtenianhypnosis.com
Although open to anyone interested in this fascinating hypnosis modality, this website information is for graduates of the Hypnotism Training Institute of Alberta.

http://www.connectwithanny.com
This is the best place to keep up to date with Anny – including seeing all her latest books and how to order them on Amazon.

Other Books By Anny Slegten…

REIKI PURE AND SIMPLE

Volume I: The Sacred Rites

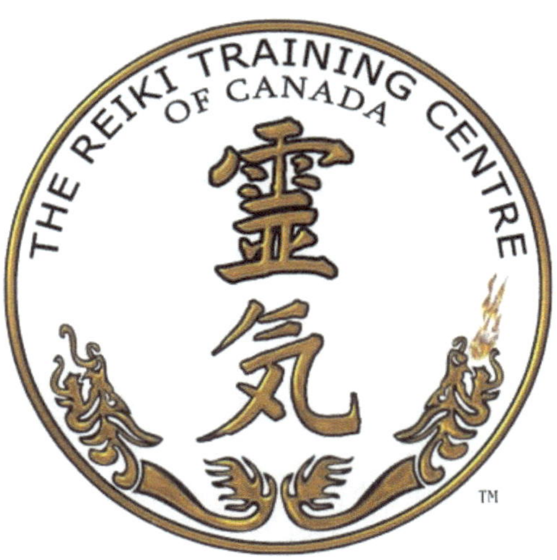

Anny J. Slegten

Reiki Training Centre of Canada
Class Material
http://www.reiki-canada.com

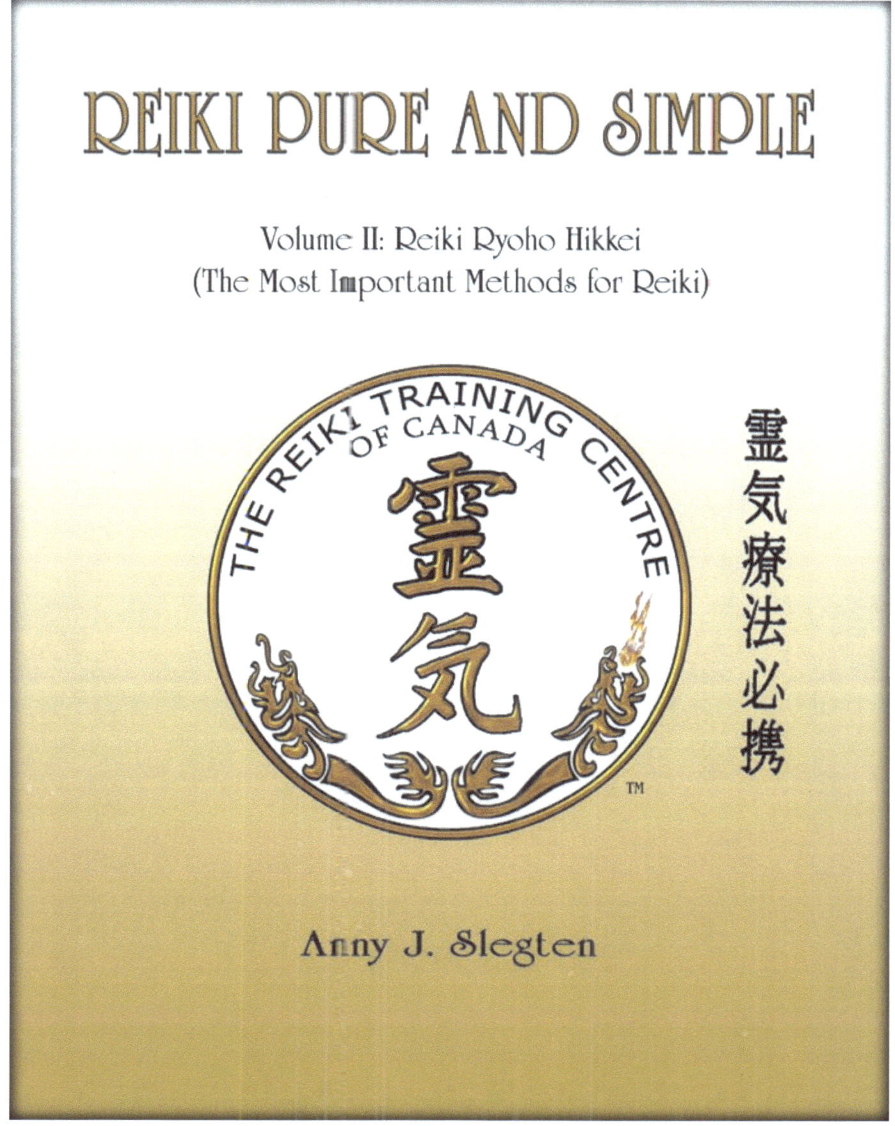

This book is a must read for Reiki Practitioners
regardless of their spiritual lineage
and could be of great benefit to Energy Healers
http://www.reiki-canada.com

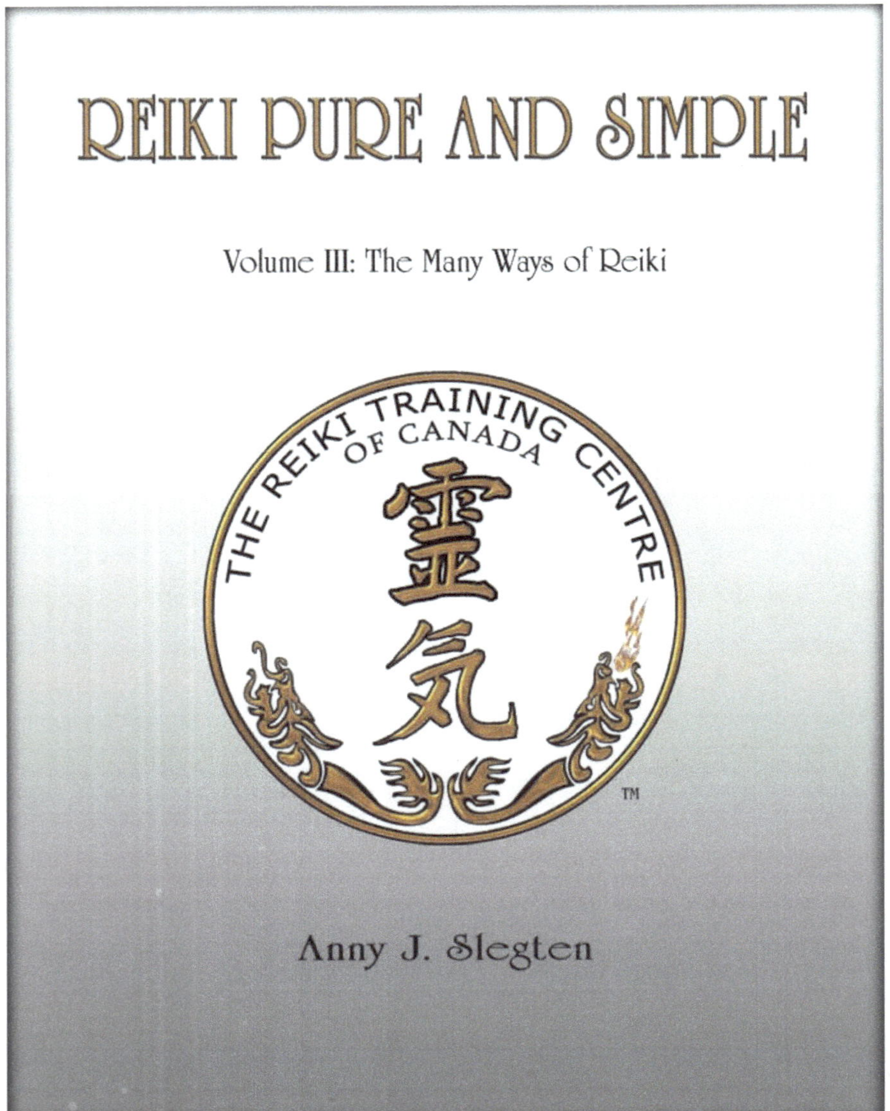

The Many Ways of Reiki
http://www.reiki-canada.com

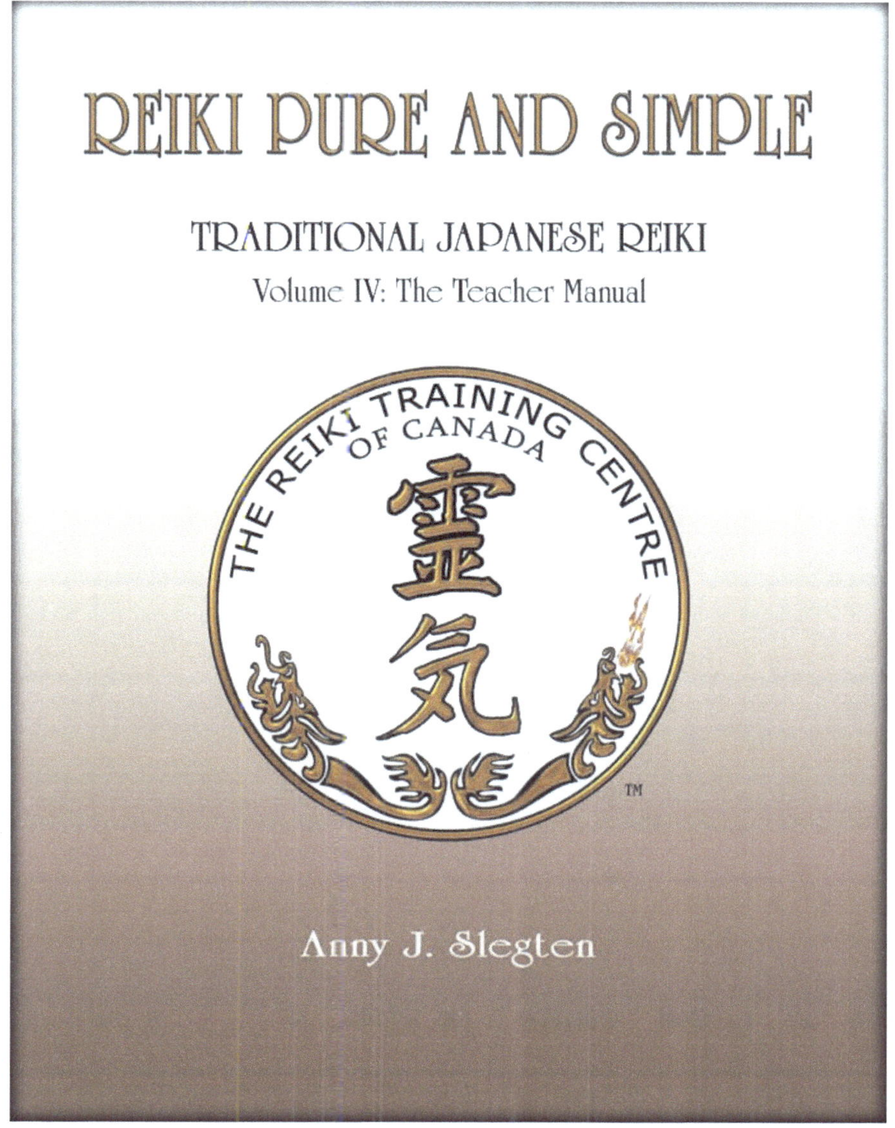

The Reiki Training Centre of Canada
Teacher's Manual
http://www.reiki-canada.com

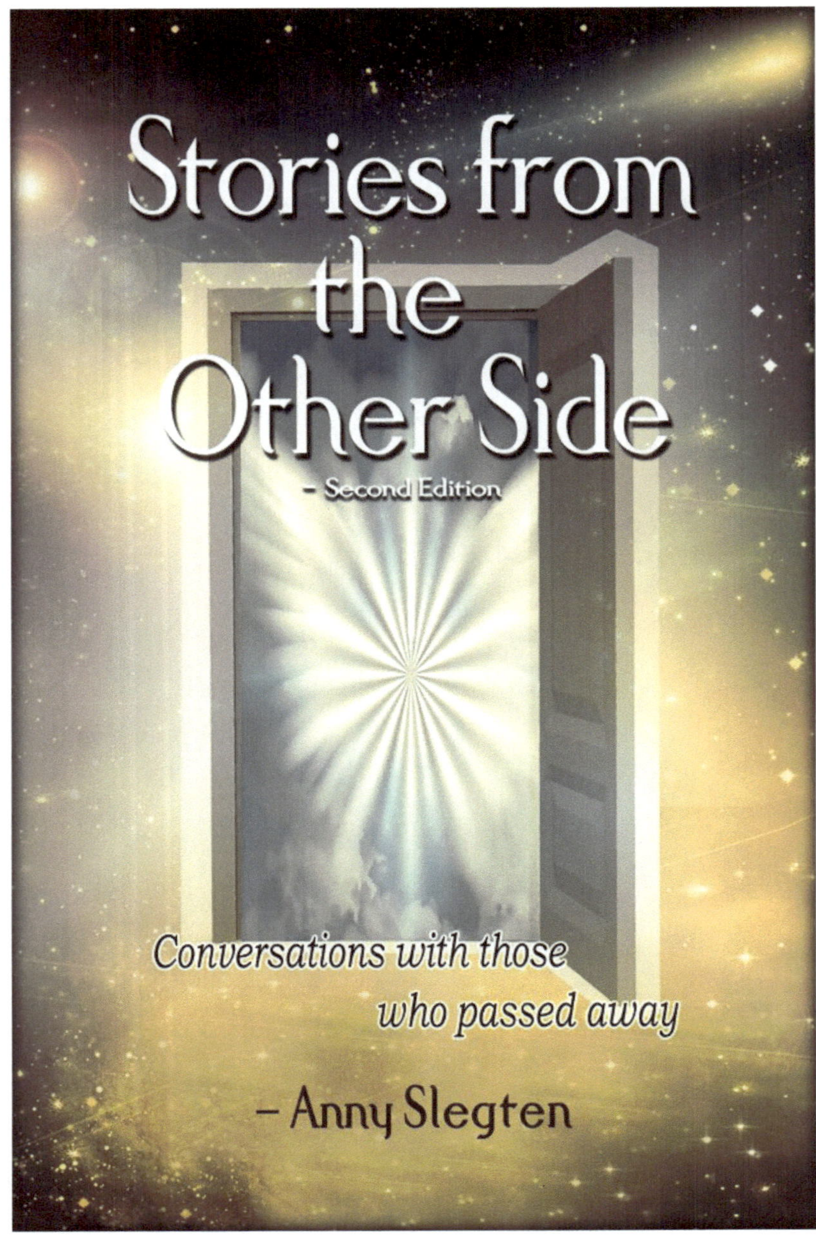

Stories from The Other Side – Second Edition
http://www.connectwithanny.com

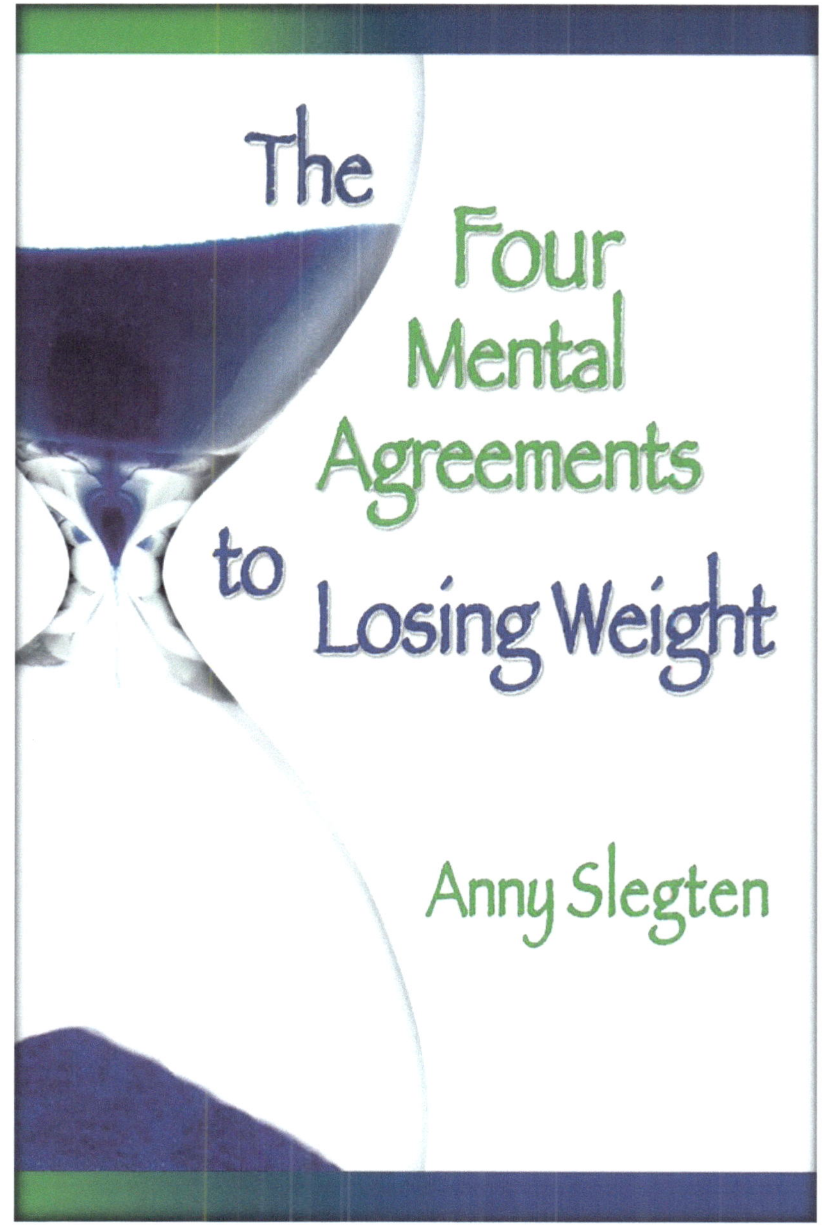

The Four Mental Agreements
To Losing Weight
http://www.connectwithanny.com

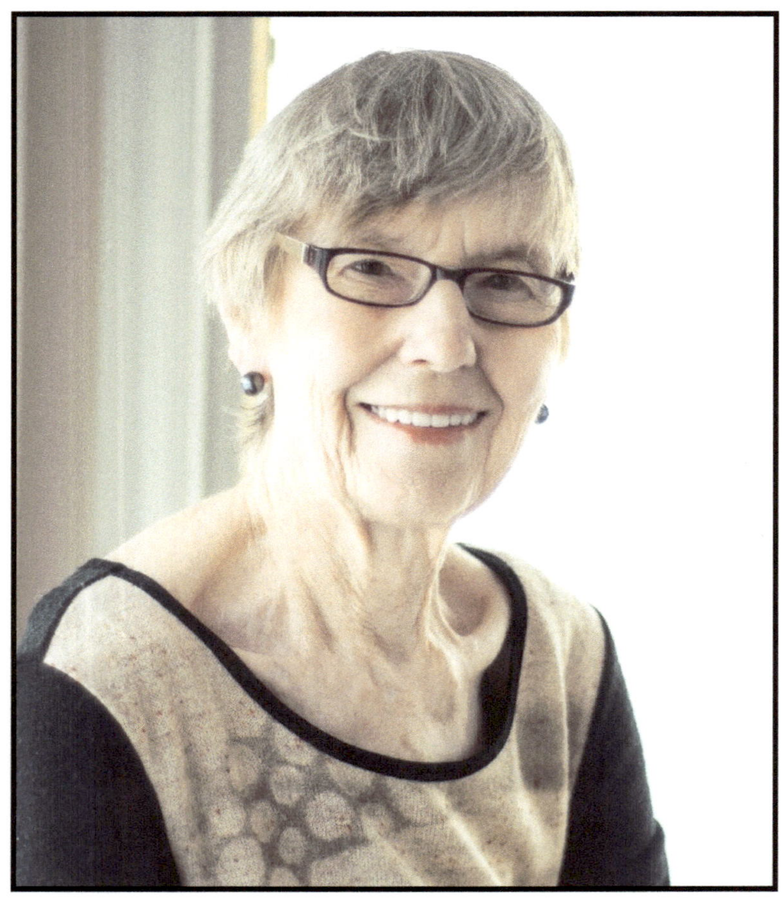

About The Author

As Director of The Hypnotism Training Institute of Alberta and The Reiki Training Centre of Canada, Anny has developed and structured the training and curriculum to the highest standards for both The Hypnotism Training Institute of Alberta and the Reiki Training Centre of Canada.

She offers training to students that come from all over Canada and around the world.

Anny has experienced and lived in many corners of the globe and this has given her a unique understanding of many cultures.

Anny's Belgian parents were from the Flemish part of Belgium and were speaking Flemish (Dutch) at home. Living in Congo, everything was in French.

Although she never spoke Flemish (Dutch), Anny speaks English with a guttural Dutch/German accent. Living in the English-speaking part of Canada for decades, Anny now speaks French with an English accent!

Anny is an Author and holds certifications as:

Master Hypnotist
Clinical Hypnotherapist
Hypno-Baby Birthing Facilitator and Instructor
HypnoBirthing™ Fertility Therapist for Men & Women
Reiki Master/Teacher
Master Remote Viewer

Anny is a world renowned Clinical Hypnotherapist and Hypnologist in full time practice since 1984 as well as a Hypno-Energy worker since 2008.

In 1986 Anny created and developed an unique method using hypnosis for distance services - Virtual Sessions.

Over the years these Virtual Sessions proved to be an effective, useful, and efficient method for investigations and putting closure on both present and past issues - resulting in peace of mind.

To know more about Anny, please visit www.annyslegten.com and make sure to read what she published on her Blog.

Do you wonder what else Anny is publishing?

Visit www.connectwithanny.com

www.ingramcontent.com/pod-product-compliance
Lightning Source LLC
Chambersburg PA
CBHW050813220326
41598CB00006B/200

* 9 7 8 1 7 7 5 2 4 8 9 8 9 *